TONY DEARING

I WANT MY MIND BACK

The Go Cogno Approach to Halt or Reverse Mild Cognitive Impairment

D1707754

The author is not a medical professional and this book does not offer medical advice. It is intended for informational purposes only, and is not a substitute for the medical opinion, diagnosis and treatment you should secure from a doctor, ideally one who specializes in cognition. Never make changes that can affect your health without first consulting a doctor, and always strive to work in tandem with your doctor as partners in brain health. The author shall not be liable or responsible for any loss or damage allegedly arising from any information in this book.

First edition

This book was professionally typeset on Reedsy.
Find out more at reedsy.com

To Carla R. Dearing, devoted mother, distinguished businesswoman and tireless community servant. Every word I write about brain health and the defense of cognition is offered in loving memory of her.

"A great deal of fear is a result of just not knowing. We do not know what is involved in a new situation. We do not know whether we can deal with it. The sooner we learn what it entails, the sooner we can dissolve our fear."

— Eleanor Roosevelt

Contents

Foreword

This is a very exciting time to be working in the field of neuroscience and neurodegenerative diseases. Some of us believe we are witnessing the dawn of the age of treatable neurodegenerative diseases like Alzheimer's, Parkinson's, Lewy Body Disease and others. For many of us, mild cognitive impairment (MCI) is the first alarm bell of an impending neurodegenerative disease. Medical research tells us that by the time someone has developed MCI, there is already quite a bit of "brain damage" that has set in.

But that is not the end of the story. Prior to 2014, very few people were hopeful about trying to halt or reverse neurodegeneration. Billions and billions of dollars spent on drug trials had, thus far, been failures. Individuals with cognitive impairment were essentially left with very little hope of improvement. However, our collective clinical experience and now more and more emerging research suggests that there are many things that can be done to slow, halt, or even improve cognitive decline.

Take that in for a minute . . . as of 2020 there are several things you can do to impact and improve cognitive decline. This is revolutionary.

While large academic centers are doing the heavy lifting of running clinical trials, individuals and smaller organizations are already bringing this critical information to individuals in dire need of solutions.

Tony Dearing's book, "I Want My Mind Back," summarizes and guides you through so much of this revolutionary information.

The hard truth is, however, that improvement takes work. If you think you will find a few pills that are going to turn all your cognitive symptoms around I am sorry to say that is simply not the case.

Continuing to live your life in the same manner that caused you to develop cognitive impairment will obviously not give rise to improvements.

But if you are willing to take a hard look at the factors in life that drive wellness and have the ability to create powerful metabolic and epigenetic changes, there is hope for you and for all of us impacted by these devastating neurodegenerative diseases.

Critical factors to examine include:

- Nutrition
- Movement
- Sleep quality
- Management of Stress
- Cognitive Training
- Awareness of environmental toxins (such as mercury) that Tony has included a chapter on.

It's important to mention the many personal stories that Tony shares with you, supporting this information. Data is great, but the practical implementation of the data is where a lot of folks get tripped up. Being part of support groups can make all the difference in our ability to carry out the recommendations and succeed in pushing back against MCI and other forms of cognitive decline.

Thank you for all the great work you are doing, Tony!

Nate Bergman DO
  Chief Scientific Wellness Officer
  Kemper Cognitive Wellness
  Cleveland, Ohio
  November 2020

CHAPTER 1 — The Go Cogno Approach

MIRIAM DIDN'T start out seeing herself as someone who could beat mild cognitive impairment. That didn't even seem like a possibility to her.

But early one day in September 2019, she logged into a support group on Facebook to share the good news.

Here's exactly how she put it:

> *Good morning, everyone! I'm so happy to have been a part of this group while living with mild cognitive impairment for the past 4 or more years.*
>
> *I'm very ecstatic to report, after visiting my Neurologist yesterday, I have experienced a complete reversal due to adherence to a very strict diet, vigorous cardiovascular exercise, reduction of stress, and practice of mindfulness techniques.*
>
> *Thank you for being such a wonderful, supportive group and I wish everyone the best!*

It was a startling, inspiring declaration that seemed to come out of nowhere.

Miriam hadn't posted to our Facebook group for quite a while, and the last time we heard from her, she sounded like anyone else facing this ominous condition. Frightened. Overwhelmed. Groping for answers.

Yet here she was, announcing that she had reversed her cognitive loss, and sounding downright giddy about it.

To the members of our Facebook group, that felt like a miracle. If only they could halt or reverse their own MCI, the way Miriam had. That was their dream, too. The congratulations came in ALL CAPS with a flurry of exclamation points.

> *"FANTASTIC!!! So happy for you."*
>
> *"Wonderful news and so glad that you shared it. You give us HOPE!"*
>
> *"OMG!! So happy for you!!! Can you share the strict diet? And mindfulness techniques? Trying to help my LO every day!!!"*

There is a reason I share this story, and it's not because I want you to meet Miriam.

It's because I want you to be Miriam.

What she did is entirely possible for you. And she'd be the first to tell you that.

"When I started on this journey of recovery, my goal was to keep myself from getting worse; that's all I wanted," Miriam says. "But what happened was, I got better and it reversed, and I wasn't expecting that. I want people to know if that happened to me, it could happen to you."

MY MISSION: TO GIVE YOU HOPE AND A PATH

What if it could happen for you? What if it did? Would that be a miracle?

The answer is, it wouldn't. What Miriam accomplished wasn't miraculous at all. It's becoming more common every day. Thanks to revolutionary advances in research and a whole new array of cutting-edge treatments, it is now quite possible to slow, halt or reverse cognitive decline when caught at the MCI stage.

For Miriam, for you, for anyone with mild cognitive impairment, these breakthroughs offer hope, something people with MCI desperately need.

And they offer a way, the other thing so many people facing this vague, baffling diagnosis so often find themselves without.

That, then, is my mission: To give you hope and a path. To invite you to Go Cogno.

To Go Cogno is to become an advocate for your own care and the architect of your own actions. It's based on a set of best practices that I arrived at over a period of years spent talking to really smart doctors who are finding new, effective ways to treat cognitive impairment and the patients who are gamely battling MCI and prevailing against it.

It's not a magic formula. It's not a proprietary protocol. Rather, it is an approach I have seen work again and again for real people in the real world as they took aggressive steps to defend their cognition.

They're the ones who had the resolve to act and the resourcefulness to succeed, and they deserve the credit. All I've done is distill their successes into a clear and easy-to-follow course of action that shows you how possible it becomes to halt or reverse your cognitive loss when you

- get a diagnosis you understand and can act on;
- find yourself the quality of care that everyone with MCI deserves, but many go without;
- own your version of MCI, because you're the only one who has it;
- commit to the five lifestyle essentials that pave the way to better brain health;
- defend your brain against the cognitive peril of such toxins as mercury, arsenic or mold; and
- enroll in a clinical trial if that's an option for you.

NEW AND NOVEL TREATMENTS FOR MCI

If you're reading this book, I assume you either have been diagnosed with mild cognitive impairment, or you have a loved one with MCI. Or at the very least, you may be experiencing memory problems so worrisome that you presume it's some form of neurological impairment, even if you don't know and you're afraid to find out.

So let me assure you, not at all facetiously, that there's never been a better time to be diagnosed with MCI.

Even a few short years ago, the treatment options for mild cognitive impairment were meager to nonexistent. It generally went like this: The doctor gave the diagnosis, shrugged and said, "There's not much we can do for you. Come back and see me in a year."

The poor patient went home baffled and terrified. *Mild cognitive impairment? Never heard of it. I don't know anyone else who has it. Am I the only one? Why me? What did I ever do to deserve this?*

A Google search did nothing to ease that sense of alarm and dread. There was scant information available online, and it tended to be outdated and inaccurate, referring to MCI as "incipient dementia" and projecting that 80 percent of the people who had it would progress to Alzheimer's in fairly short order.

This misguided belief — that mild cognitive impairment almost surely means dementia and there's little to be done about it — has always been a profound disservice to people with MCI, and never more than now, when we know so much better.

Regardless of what you've heard, regardless of what you've read, regardless of what you fear during your darkest moments, please know this. You are not doomed by this diagnosis.

Cognitive impairment, when caught early enough, can be slowed, halted or even reversed.

I don't say this to make you feel better or to give you false hope. It is empirically true.

In this book, I will show you new scientific evidence that offers real hope. Groundbreaking research says that nearly 90 percent of people with MCI can stabilize or reverse their cognitive loss over a period of four to five years, and relatively few (approximately 12%) will progress to dementia during that time.

I will share with you the results of study after study in which thousands of people with MCI, people just like you, were shown to halt or reverse their cognitive decline through exercise, diet, meditation or brain training. When you combine healthy habits like these, the results become even more impressive.

I will introduce you to respected medical professionals who are flipping the script on mild cognitive impairment. These outspoken experts reject the gloomy prognostications of the past, when it was taboo to even hint that MCI might be halted or — heresy of heresies — to suggest that Alzheimer's disease is preventable.

They say exactly that, right out loud. They are here to tell you that cognitive impairment is treatable and reversible and they're demonstrating it by the results they see with their patients.

REAL PEOPLE, REAL RESULTS

It's not just the patients at a handful of elite, specialized MCI clinics who are getting these results.

I regularly encounter people with MCI who have experienced improvement in their cognition or at least stabilized it, often for very long periods. Does that surprise you? It surprised them, too.

Typically, these people have a history of Alzheimer's in their family and began with the assumption that their fate was sealed. In some cases, when their memory began to fail and they went to the doctor, the initial diagnosis was Alzheimer's. Their doctor prepared them for the worst. But the worst didn't come.

Instead, a year later or maybe two years later, they tested better. Their memory scores improved, or at least stopped declining. Their diagnosis was downgraded to MCI, and their cognition went on to remain stable or, better yet, eventually reverted to normal.

Remarkable as that may seem, they went about it in the most unremarkable ways.

They set out on a mission to defend their cognition, managed to do a lot of things right along the way, and got a better result than they dared to hope for.

And here's what you can take heart in: What they did is available to anyone with MCI, including you. But that effort must begin with a basic understanding of what mild cognitive impairment is, what it means to have it, and what it takes to address it.

Far too many people diagnosed with MCI are still being sent home without even the slightest grasp of that. So here, in a nutshell, is what I've learned from scores of top doctors and scientist who devote themselves to mild cognitive impairment.

MCI is not a specific disease. It's more of a catchall term, a way for your doctor to describe a degree of cognitive loss that's unusual for someone your age. (For a more detailed look at MCI, see the FAQ in the Appendix.)

MCI isn't a form of dementia, and it doesn't mean you're going to get dementia, although it puts you at higher risk.

About half of people with MCI will see their memory loss stabilize for a period of four to five years after their diagnosis. Another third or so will return to cognitively normal.

So that outdated information you found on the Internet saying 80 percent of people with MCI will progress to dementia over five years? It's way off the mark. In actuality, maybe 10 to 12 percent of people with MCI will progress to dementia over that amount of time.

So the odds of slowing or stabilizing cognitive decline at the MCI stage are actually pretty good, and whatever your odds, they become even better when you Go Cogno.

AN EXERCISE IN 'COGNITIVE ORIENTEERING'

For sure, the Go Cogno approach is infused with what I've learned from the leading experts on MCI. There are so many brilliant, amazing people working on MCI these days. They are helping us get a better handle on what mild cognitive impairment is, what it's doing to your brain, and what you can do to defend yourself against it.

They've provided us with the pillars of brain health, and they have given us the ability to say with confidence, yes, you can potentially slow, halt or reverse this thing.

Go Cogno is entirely consistent with the pedagogy of these experts. But it goes one important step further. It shows you how to take that knowledge, go out into the real world, and make it work for you.

I say this because Go Cogno is, in essence, a crowd-sourced approach. It is of, for and by people with MCI. Because they are the ones out there doing this. And Go Cogno is how they did it.

When you've had a chance to interact with hundreds of people who have MCI, and you see the ones who are succeeding, and getting the results other people aren't, you naturally wonder why. What are these people doing right? What's working for them?

So I started asking. The more people I talked to, the clearer the pattern became. Over and over again, I kept seeing the same set

7

of commonalities in the way these people defended their cognition. Eventually, that coalesced into the Go Cogno approach.

Nobody can promise you the results these people got. But nobody promised them those results either. They just went out and did it. What they've been fortunate enough to achieve, I want to make every bit as available to you.

In the chapters that follow, we will arm you with what you need to know — and do — in order to defend your cognition. But don't expect some GPS-style solution that maps out the exact route to your final destination. This is more directional.

Are you familiar with orienteering? It's a sport where the competitors are given a compass and a basic topographical map and use those to traverse through unfamiliar terrain. They're all trying to get to the same place, but no two of them take the same route. Each has to find his or her own way.

That's what this is. Cognitive orienteering. It's designed to point you in the right direction and provide guideposts along the way as you get from where you are now to a cognitively better place.

I wish this book didn't need to exist. I wish every person with MCI walked out of the doctor's office with a firm grasp of their diagnosis, a clear and aggressive course of treatment and some degree of confidence that they can indeed slow, halt or reverse the symptoms they're experiencing.

Someday, that will be true for everyone.

For now, let's make it true for you, by using the Go Cogno approach to help guide you there.

Fortunately, this is not something you have to figure out entirely for yourself. You are following in the footsteps of those who've come before you.

People like Miriam, and so many others.

Their outcome is now your opportunity — as long as you commit to better brain health and are willing to put in the work.

As Václav Havel once said:

"It is not enough to stare up the steps. We must step up the stairs."

Are you ready to take that first step?

Then let's Go Cogno. Your journey begins when you turn the page.

TAKEAWAYS FROM CHAPTER 1

You are not doomed by your diagnosis. It is possible to slow, halt or reverse MCI and the odds of doing so are actually good.

To Go Cogno is to be an advocate for your own care and the architect of your own actions. It's a set of best practices gleaned from dedicated doctors who are pioneering new treatments and the patients who gamely battle MCI and prevail against it.

The Go Cogno approach has worked for real people in the real world. They set out to defend their cognition, managed to do a lot of things right, and got a better result than they dared to hope for.

No one can promise you the results that others got, but no one promised them those results either. Their outcome is now your opportunity — as long as you commit to better brain health and are willing to put in the work.

ONE ACTION, RIGHT NOW: Turn to Chapter 2

CHAPTER 2 — A Diagnosis To Act On

IT BEGINS with "subjective memory concerns."

That's what doctors call it when you can tell something's gone wrong in your brain and it scares the hell out of you.

If you have MCI, you know how harrowing it can be when the mind begins to fail.

You walk into a room and can't remember why you went there. Someone tells you something, and five minutes later, you have to ask again. You were always a whiz with numbers, but now you can't balance your checkbook. You look at your grandchildren and don't know their names.

You might be able to dismiss or hide these scary signs for a while, but they persist. Finally, you have to face the truth. There's something seriously wrong with your mind and you need to see a doctor about it.

For anyone with MCI, that is the crucial move. Because the problem begins when you notice it. But the solution doesn't begin until you get a diagnosis.

That diagnosis represents the first, most fundamental step in confronting your MCI. You want to walk out of the doctor's office with a diagnosis you understand, accept and can act upon.

If that's what you've got, you're one of the lucky few.

Based on my experiences with the thousands of people who come to my website, GoCogno.com, or watch my weekly brain health videos on

YouTube, I would say MCI remains one of the more widely misunder-stood and misdiagnosed conditions in medicine.

I deal with people every day who have been to a doctor and have received a diagnosis, yet they still have little grasp of what they are dealing with or how to address it. And that puts them at such a disadvantage.

Know thy enemy, right?

What Sun Tzu actually said was:

> *"If you know neither the enemy nor yourself, you will succumb in every battle."*

So please know this: The journey ahead is about more than eating blueberries or hitting the gym. It's an exercise in personal growth. It will call upon you to go to a place of greater self-awareness and deeper understanding. Because the better you come to know MCI, and the better you come to know your own strengths and vulnerabilities, the more likely you are to get the result you desire.

And that begins with a proper diagnosis. So let's make sure you have one — or help you get one.

Use this as the litmus test:

> *"I have a diagnosis that I understand, accept and am ready to act on."*

If you can answer that with a yes, good for you. You've got what you need to get started and you're welcome to skip ahead to Chapter 3.

If the answer is no, then let's unpack that and see what might have gone wrong.

Maybe you have a diagnosis, but you don't understand it. Or you doubt your diagnosis. Or maybe you haven't gotten a diagnosis yet. Let's look more closely at each of those scenarios.

SCENARIO 1 — I DON'T HAVE A DIAGNOSIS YET

If you've been to a doctor, but you're still waiting to see a specialist for your diagnosis, that time in between can be agonizing. But you're moving in the right direction, and in the meantime, you can still get a lot out of this book. There's plenty you can do even now to defend your cognition and get a head start on whatever your diagnosis turns out to be.

If you haven't been to the doctor yet, because you're afraid of what you might find out, then I am required to give you what Ann Landers called the "20 lashes with a wet spaghetti noodle." You need to see the doctor ASAP.

Everything we know about slowing, halting or reversing cognitive impairment works better when the problem is caught as early as possible.

If you had a broken toe, you wouldn't wait six months, or a year, or three years to have it looked at. Yet that's typically how long people put off a visit to the doctor after they first begin to notice signs of cognitive decline. We're not talking about your big toe here. We're talking about your brain. Please, please, please go see a doctor. Now.

SCENARIO 2 — I HAVE A DIAGNOSIS, BUT I DON'T UNDERSTAND IT

Sadly, this seems to be a recurring theme for people facing cognitive impairment. There are at least a couple of common ways I see this occur, and let's look at an example of each.

You didn't get a correct diagnosis because you weren't properly evaluated and the doctor jumped to the wrong conclusion.

Doug Thompson is a 71-year-old former newspaperman and Congressional press secretary who now lives in the Blue Ridge Mountains, where he runs a hyperlocal website called the Blue Ridge Muse.

In 2015, Thompson was diagnosed with MCI due to a head injury suffered in a motorcycle accident. That diagnosis came after a neuropsychologist gave him a careful, thorough examination that took more than three hours. There was no indication of Alzheimer's (a fact that becomes important as this story unfolds).

Thompson learned to accept his MCI and live with it, and stays active and productive. But like a lot of people with MCI, he had a constant urge to know how he was doing. Was his cognition getting any better? Had it gotten worse? So in April 2019, four years after his initial diagnosis, he went to his family doctor and asked to be tested again.

This time, he was sent to a neurologist, where he had a nightmarish experience that he ended up chronicling on his website.

The cognitive testing, if you can call it that, was perfunctory. The neurologist asked him five simple questions, including "What year is this?" and "Where do you live?" Thompson only got one answer wrong. The neurologist then handed him a prescription for Aricept, with no explanation other than "it's something that might help you remember things." That was it. Thompson was in and out of the neurologist's office in less than 20 minutes.

Thompson went home, took the medicine, and immediately began experiencing severe side effects. He couldn't sleep. He suffered muscle cramps that left him unable to walk, drive or do any productive work. He knew something was seriously wrong.

Thompson looked Aricept up online and discovered it's a medication prescribed to people with mild to moderate Alzheimer's.(*) He stopped taking it, and his symptoms quickly improved. He sent the neurologist a note saying he'd quit his medication and didn't want any other medicine of that sort.

Instead of talking to him or bringing him in for further evaluation, the neurologist wrote Thompson a new prescription, this time for Namenda, a drug for patients with moderate to severe Alzheimer's.

Thompson knew better than to continue down that road. He ditched the neurologist, went back to his primary care doctor and asked to be referred to the neuropsychologist's office where he was originally diagnosed. "They tested and treated me before," he said. "They know me."

Chalk it up to a lesson learned the hard way. I wish I could tell you this is a rare occurrence, but it's not. It actually happens quite often. So does the next scenario we're going to explore.

You got a diagnosis, but the doctor didn't take the time to really explain it to you.

Dolores could tell it wasn't going to go well from the moment she arrived at the doctor's office. Her test results were back and she was there to receive her diagnosis. "You don't have an appointment," they told her. She insisted she did. They told her to take a seat in the waiting room.

Half an hour later, a nurse approached Dolores. "Sorry," the nurse said. "It looks like you and another patient were booked for the same time. We'll let you know when the doctor can see you."

After another hour of waiting, her name was called. Dolores was supposed to have 30 minutes with the doctor, but because of the double booking, the nurse said they were running behind and would have to shorten her visit. After waiting two hours, she got barely 15 minutes with the doctor.

The doctor handed Dolores some paperwork but didn't say anything about her diagnosis. The discussion was vague and curt, and then the doctor excused himself and was off to his next patient. Dolores and her husband left the office with nothing but unanswered questions.

When she got home, she went through the papers they'd given her. Her diagnosis was listed as "pseudo-dementia." Pseudo-what? Dolores had no idea what she was dealing with. The doctor had not even mentioned that word, let alone explained it to her.

Pseudo-dementia is a term that's been around since the 1960s and is intended to describe dementia-like symptoms associated with depression. Not that Dolores knew that. Her visit to the neurologist had left her completely in the dark. She showed up in our Facebook group asking if anyone knew what pseudo-dementia was.

That is so often what passes for patient education in the world of MCI these days. People who didn't get a good explanation from their doctor reaching out to other people with MCI who don't have answers to their own questions, let alone someone else's.

WHAT A PROPER DIAGNOSIS LOOKS LIKE

Does either of those scenarios sound familiar to you? How would you describe your own experience so far? Has it been a good one? Or a horror story? Or somewhere in between?

If the diagnosis and care you have right now is less than satisfactory, don't despair. Don't give up on the medical system. And don't give up on yourself. Good care exists in the world of MCI today. You just haven't found it yet.

There are good doctors out there who know all the steps they're supposed to take. Who know how to test you properly. Who know how to interpret those results and arrive at an appropriate diagnosis, and then explain that diagnosis to you in a way you understand, and answer your questions and offer you encouragement and support and a way forward.

None of that is too much to ask. And every bit of it is essential as you set out to defend your cognition.

When I look at people I have seen successfully slow, halt or reverse their MCI, the first thing they have in common is the quality of their diagnosis, which allowed them to understand what they were dealing with and how to address it.

To Go Cogno is to become an advocate for your own care and the architect of your own actions. If you don't have confidence in your diagnosis — or in your doctor, for that matter — that is a time when it becomes absolutely essential for you to advocate for yourself.

You deserve to know all the steps a doctor is supposed to take in evaluating you for MCI, and to ask for something you didn't get if the doctor missed a step. (To learn what the proper steps are, see the Diagnosis Checklist in Appendix B.)

You deserve to know the name of any cognitive test you were given, what your score was, and what that score means.

You have a right to reflect on what you don't understand about your diagnosis, make a list of questions, bring them with you to your next appointment, and get them answered.

You may ask to see a specialist in MCI if you haven't been referred to one.

You are allowed to seek a second opinion if you doubt your diagnosis.

Only you know what you don't know, and advocating for yourself is how you fill the gaps in your understanding. Keep asking questions until you're satisfied with the answers you're getting.

ACCEPTING THE AMBIGUITY OF MCI

Because mild cognitive impairment is an incredibly complex, multi-faceted condition, the answers may not be as exact as you want them to be. There's a certain amount of ambiguity you may have to be willing to accept.

When I was 60, I was running on a treadmill and felt a "pop" in my foot. The pain was excruciating. I went to the Urgent Care, where they asked me some questions and took an X-ray. Then the doctor came in to speak with me.

"You've got a stress fracture in your foot," he said. "It's so small it didn't even show up on the X-ray, but we can tell that's what it is." He prescribed me pain pills, gave me a boot to wear and told me the fracture would heal itself in a month or so.

That is what our medical system is designed to do well, and what we have been trained to want from it. The all-knowing doctor tells you precisely what's wrong, gives you a pill, and you get better.

MCI doesn't lend itself to that. It can be caused by a seemingly infinite number of things, and often it's a Gordian combination of causes. Many people with MCI also have other chronic medical conditions, and that further complicates the matter. It becomes hard to tell what's causing what.

In some cases, there's an obvious cause. If you have a Vitamin B12 deficiency, that all by itself can result in cognitive impairment serious enough to be mistaken for dementia. A B12 deficiency is easy to detect and easy to treat, and the cognitive problems go away.

In most cases, it's not so obvious. There's still a lot we don't know about the human brain and cognition, but we know enough for doctors to give you a thorough examination and figure out what's likely to have gone wrong. Maybe not with exactitude, but with enough clarity to suggest a course of treatment.

Whatever that level of clarity is, don't let the doctors hoard it. You need clarity too, and you have a right to ask. At the very least, you want to understand what your diagnosis is and why the doctors think that's the correct diagnosis for you.

MCI CAN BE "DUE TO" MYRIAD CAUSES

Ideally, your diagnosis should include a "due to." Not "You have MCI," but "You have MCI due to (doctor fills in the blank)."

Many people diagnosed with mild cognitive impairment automatically assume that their MCI is due to Alzheimer's disease, especially if Alzheimer's runs in the family.

That was certainly the case with Miriam, the woman I introduced you to at the beginning of this book.

Miriam was 50 years old, married with three adult children and employed as an accountant in Texas when her memory began to slip.

"I was working a very stressful job," she says. "The thing I remember most is that I would have to run meetings and when someone else was talking, I couldn't write down what people were saying because I couldn't remember what they said."

She wasn't the only one to notice. "At one point, my manager said,

'Miriam, they just told you that,'" she recalls. "But I couldn't write it down. It was gone. I thought, 'You didn't used to do this. Something is wrong.' I started to get really stressed out."

Miriam assumed the worst. Alzheimer's runs in her family, on both sides. "But it really threw me, because I thought it was happening too soon," she says. "It didn't hit my family until they were in their 70s, and I was 50."

Miriam's worst fear turned out to be unfounded. She talked to her doctor, who sent her for an MRI and referred her to a neuropsychologist for cognitive testing. The following month, the results came back — and it was better news than she expected. She didn't have Alzheimer's.

That's the value of an accurate diagnosis. Everyone fears Alzheimer's, and it's so easy for patients — and even doctors — to assume Alzheimer's is the underlying cause. But you'd be surprised how often it's not.

Your mild cognitive impairment is due to _____??????

Don't let your imagination fill in that blank. Get an answer, one you can act aggressively on.

Miriam assumed she had Alzheimer's, but she didn't. Her diagnosis was MCI due to vascular disease and depression. The neurologist who gave Doug Thompson a cursory exam assumed Doug had Alzheimer's, but he didn't. Thompson had MCI due to a head injury.

There are so many possible ways to end that sentence. There's MCI due to a thyroid condition. There's MCI due to Alzheimer's disease or Parkinson's disease. There's MCI due to overmedication, a sleep disorder, a vitamin deficiency, alcohol abuse, or some combination of any of the above.

Each of these is a different version of MCI, calling for a different approach to treatment.

The right treatment for you will be shaped by your diagnosis, and that shouldn't be a mystery to you.

If you don't have good answers, keep asking until you get better answers. If your doctors can't give you better answers, you may need better doctors. That's what we'll talk about next.

TAKEAWAYS FROM CHAPTER 2

The diagnosis represents the first, most fundamental step in confronting your MCI. You want to walk out of the doctor's office with a diagnosis you understand and can act upon.

If you have cognitive concerns and haven't had them checked, see a doctor now. Everything we know about slowing, halting or reversing cognitive impairment works better when the problem is caught as early as possible.

You deserve a proper, thorough evaluation and a clear explanation of what your diagnosis is and why your doctor thinks it's the correct diagnosis for you.

Ideally, your diagnosis will include a "due to." There are many things MCI may be due to, and it's often not Alzheimer's. Many of the possible causes are treatable.

You have a right to reflect on what you don't understand about your diagnosis, make a list of questions, bring them with you to your next appointment, and get them answered.

ONE ACTION, RIGHT NOW: Use the Diagnosis Checklist to see if your doctors took all the proper steps in arriving at your diagnosis.

(* Aricept is an Alzheimer's drug that is sometimes prescribed "off-label" to MCI patients. It has not been scientifically shown to reduce the progression from MCI to dementia, but some studies suggest it may help relieve symptoms in some people with MCI. It's recommended that the doctor educate the patient about this before prescribing the drug. Aricept can have serious side effects, so a doctor may choose not to prescribe it even if the patient requests it.)

CHAPTER 3 — Getting The Right Care

WHEN YOU'VE been diagnosed with MCI, you have a couple of options. You can accept whatever medical care comes your way. Or you can go out and find the best care you can get.

For you, that probably won't mean hopping on your private jet and flying off to the Mayo Clinic. But don't let that stop you. You don't necessarily have to break the bank or go to the ends of the earth to find a capable specialist who understands how to combat MCI. That expertise may be closer to home than you realized.

It's really about looking carefully at the medical care within your reach, and not accepting less than the best options available, because you've got too much at stake to settle for crapola care.

There's too much of that being foisted on people with MCI as it is.

It pains me to say that, because it makes me sound so anti-doctor. I am not out to demonize doctors or dump on the medical system. Just the opposite. I spend a lot of my time around brilliant, dedicated doctors who are passionate about helping people with MCI and who are doing amazing things and seeing good results with their patients. I have the utmost respect for them and their innovative work.

But it's hard to watch these exciting new approaches in action and not be galled by the gap between the excellent care some people with MCI get and the nearly nonexistent care others are subjected to.

Too many doctors out there are stuck in the way-back machine, and still say things like, "There's nothing we can do."

That isn't just a disservice to people with MCI. It's flat-out wrong. There's a lot they can do for you. There's a lot you can do for yourself. The right doctor can show you what those things are.

The wrong doctor won't even suggest it's a possibility.

To understand how wildly different the experience can be, depending on who your doctor is, let's look at two examples.

THE BEST OF CARE, THE WORST OF CARE

We'll start with Naomi, whose mother was diagnosed with MCI in the summer of 2019. When I first met her, here's the story she had to tell:

"My mother is 84 years old," Naomi said. "Her neurologist did not give me any information or options for what we can do to stop it, reverse it or delay it. He just said that some individuals, the symptoms stay the same or return to normal or progress. He said he had no way of knowing.

"It made me very sad and helpless that there was nothing we can do until I did some research. There is no one to ask or guide me here. The doctors don't offer any hope. I think I want to change my mom's primary doctor to a doctor in internal medicine or geriatric medicine. And I want to find a neurologist who can guide us, who believes that food is medicine."

Now let's compare that to the experience of someone with MCI who's being treated by Dr. Richard Isaacson, founder of the Alzheimer's Prevention Clinic at Weill Cornell Medicine in New York.

Back when I first met Dr. Isaacson, he was viewed warily by the medical profession. He'd gone rogue. At that time, it was not considered OK to even suggest that Alzheimer's could be prevented in a person with MCI. Yet Dr. Isaacson named his center the Alzheimer's Prevention

Clinic. He ruefully recalls the years he's spent having tradition-bound doctors "throw tomatoes at me."

Dr. Isaacson didn't listen to the doubters. He was too busy helping people with MCI fend off dementia. In October 2019, he published the results of a study showing that putting patients with MCI on a highly individualized treatment plan for 18 months led to improved scores on a combination of cognitive tests.

I wasn't surprised by these findings, partly because I'd been given a sneak preview of his results before they were published, and partly because I had seen the intensive, high-level care he was providing to patients with MCI.

If you are a patient of Dr. Isaacson, he meets with you every six months. And each time he sits down with you, he gives you a list of things he wants you to work on between then and the next session. He told me that for his typical patient, there can be anywhere from 20 to as many as 50 things on that list.

Up to fifty things. Every six months. Does that sound like "nothing" to you?

RATING YOUR DOCTOR ON THE "ALOOFNESS INDEX"

That is as stark a contrast as I can offer you between the haves and have-nots in the world of treatment for MCI.

There are Dr. Isaacson's patients, who get an intensive, individualized treatment plan. There's Naomi, whose mother wasn't offered even a glimmer of guidance or hope. And then there's you, sitting somewhere between those two extremes.

Only you can say how satisfied you are with the care you're getting from your doctor or medical team right now. But to help you take stock of that, let's do a little exercise, by filling in the blanks below. Answer Yes or No to the following statements.

The doctor I'm working with right now:

_____ Is well-versed in MCI

_____ Seems to be up on the latest treatments

_____ Communicates well, explains things, answers my questions

_____ Shows me specific ways to protect my cognition

_____ Offers hope and encouragement

_____ Makes me feel like we're working as a team

The way you just answered those questions can tell a lot, although I wouldn't expect any neurologist to get a strong Yes on every single statement. If yours does, I'd suggest you nominate them for sainthood. What should concern you is if you see a preponderance of No's.

You might call this an aloofness index. These statements reflect what people with MCI would like from a specialist. They don't necessarily reflect what a doctor is prepared to provide.

In the least desirable scenario, the doctor may have a perfunctory conversation and send the patient on their way. Or as the saying goes, "Diagnose and adios."

You may have received that kiss-off, when there is so much more that you could and should have been offered.

"THE AMAZING NEWS IS, YOU CAN IMPROVE"

The treatment of mild cognitive impairment is evolving rapidly, with notable doctors setting the pace.

In addition to Dr. Isaacson, these clinicians include: Dr. Nate Bergman, chief scientific wellness officer at Kemper Cognitive Wellness in Cleveland; Drs. Dean and Ayesha Sherzai, co-directors of the Brain

Health and Alzheimer's Prevention Program in Loma Linda, Ca.; and Dr. Mary Kay Ross, founder and CEO of the Brain Health and Research Institute in Seattle, just to name a few of the stellar ones whom I have come to know and respect.

These doctors are aggressive in their approach and bold in what they say is possible, in terms of slowing, halting or reversing MCI. They say it can be done, and they are mapping out the ways to help you do it.

Whether you have a greater genetic risk of Alzheimer's or not, there is good science to show that people with MCI who focus on the right things — including diet, exercise, sleep, stress reduction, and brain training — can alter the course of their cognition.

"You can improve. The amazing, amazing news is that you can improve," says Dr. Nate Bergman, an internist/geriatrician trained in functional medicine and host of the Evolving Past Alzheimer's podcast. "There is so much to do, and you can get so much better. There are so many things that can happen to drive wellness."

But there is a key to making that happen. You want to catch it early, ideally at the MCI stage or sooner, and then act aggressively in defense of your cognition.

"The earlier we identify it, the more treatable it is," Dr. Bergman says. "You can do something for everybody at every stage, but in terms of reversibility or really having a remission of symptoms, it seems that you have to get this earlier. Mild cognitive impairment is a perfect time to be taking major action."

That's what the experts tell us, and that's what the most recent scientific findings confirm. I read this research copiously, and it's compelling. What persuades me even more are the real people with MCI whom I see using that information to stabilize their memory loss for very long periods of time or even reverse it.

When I talk to people who've had success in halting or reversing their MCI, I ask them how they did it. And here's one thing they invariably tell me. They didn't do it on their own. They had good medical care and took full advantage of it.

In most cases, they found that care close to home. Chances are, you can too.

Maybe you already have. If you've landed in the hands of a good neurologist, I'm happy for you. That puts you so much further ahead in the game.

But if the right care hasn't found you, then I encourage you to find it.

HOW TO FIND A GOOD SPECIALIST IN YOUR AREA

To Go Cogno is to be an advocate for your own care and the architect of your own actions. If you don't feel good about the care you're receiving, this is one of those times when you need to advocate fiercely for yourself.

Don't settle. Do some homework. Ask around. Hunt for the best neurologist or medical team you can find.

These days, it's really not any different than looking for any other form of professional help. If you needed an attorney or an accountant, you'd go about that through some combination of online research and word-of-mouth recommendations. The same applies here.

U.S. News & World Report offers a rating of the "Best Hospitals for Neurology & Neurosurgery" and you can find that here.

Another way to find a top specialist is to check the listing of medical centers and clinics that belong to what's called the Global Alzheimer's Platform Foundation, a network of progressive, cutting-edge research centers in neurology. Depending on what part of the United States or Canada you live in, one of these centers may be near you. (We'll talk much more about GAP-Net in Chapter 15.)

Referrals and word-of-mouth can be equally valuable.

As primary care doctors see more older patients with memory loss, some have a better understanding of what they're dealing with and are getting plugged into neurological resources in their area. If your GP is one of them, they may be able to give you a good referral. That's ideal, when it happens.

There are memory cafes springing up in communities, and support groups. Getting involved in one of those can be a good way to meet people who know a good neurologist they can recommend.

There's probably an Alzheimer's walk-a-thon in your area. Taking part in that is not only a positive and proactive way to help advance research, it also represents another opportunity to network with people who can help point you to a well-regarded doctor.

Here's one other tip: Visit the website of the Alzheimer's organization chapter in your state, and go to the page where they list their community education events. Check past or upcoming events, and find the name of a neurologist or neuropsychologist who puts on programs for the public. That's the kind of doctor who's going to be both knowledgeable and patient-minded. Attending one of those sessions can give you a good feel for the doctor, and if you like them and what they have to say, you can call their office and ask for an appointment.

At the very least, I hope I've given you a starting point. Combining these suggestions with your own resourcefulness can help get you to the doctor you're looking for. Whatever effort you invest in finding that doctor, it will be time well spent.

MCI can be an incredibly complex medical condition, but we understand it so much better now. We've learned ways to treat it effectively. Some people are getting that treatment; others aren't. Way too many people with MCI still find themselves stranded on an island of inadequate care.

What I hate to hear are stories like this one from Carmen, who has just come back from an appointment with her new neurologist and felt a need to unload in our Facebook group:

> *"I am just beyond aggravated. My neurologist left the state so I get assigned another one. Six months later, I went to see him today and all he was worried about was my headaches. He never asked about my memory and when I kept trying to bring it up, he would just say, "Let's check your B12. And see you back in six months." And then he left the room. . Thanks for letting me vent. Some doctors just don't give a crap."*

Sadly, some don't.

But some do. Your job is to find one who does.

TAKEAWAYS FROM CHAPTER 3

You don't have to break the bank or go to the ends of the earth to find a capable specialist who understands how to treat MCI. That expertise may be closer to home than you realized.

There's a lot a good doctor can do for you, and there's a lot you can do for yourself. The right doctor can show you what those things are.

If you don't feel good about your care, this is one of those times when you need to advocate fiercely for yourself. Don't settle. Do some homework. Ask around.

ONE ACTION, RIGHT NOW: Use the GAP-Net locater tool to search for a cutting-edge neurology center or clinic near you.

CHAPTER 4 — Owning Your Version of MCI

ONE OF the great frustrations of cognitive impairment is being told there's something you should do, when you're already doing it, and you ended up with MCI anyway.

I did an article on the brain benefits of coffee, and a commenter shot back at me with this: "Yeah, I drank three cups a day for years. A lot of good that did me."

Or there was the time I wrote about a study showing people who speak a second language are at lower risk of cognitive decline. A reader emailed me to say: "I speak five languages, and I still got MCI."

I recall a woman in particular who'd been lectured one too many times on the do's and don'ts of brain health and offered this lament:

> *"I was already doing difficult crosswords, learning a new language, interacting with others and eating healthy before my diagnosis. It drives me crazy when they tell me to do things I've already been doing. What else can I do, for Pete's sake?"*

Put a hundred people with MCI in a room, and they've all asked that question at some point. "What else can I do?"

For every one of them, the answer would be different.

You can't escape your uniqueness. No two people are the same and no two treatments for mild cognitive impairment can be the same.

Your best opportunity for slowing, halting or reversing MCI lies in an approach that's tailored to you.

In short, you need to own your version of MCI.

It's not necessarily that complicated of a thing to achieve. It's about

- recognizing your strengths, and capitalizing on what you're already doing right,
- then identifying your vulnerabilities, and shoring up the areas where your defenses are down.

If you've been sedentary for the past 20 years, or if a hectic life leaves you dining on fast food or TV dinners every night, those are glaring risk factors. If you make the effort to be more physically active and clean up your diet, you give yourself a decent chance of seeing your cognition improve.

THE OPEN "DOORS" AND "WINDOWS"

But what if you've been exercising and eating right, and MCI still weaseled its way into your brain? That feels downright unfair.

Well, MCI doesn't play fair. So rather than cursing the injustice of it all, try this instead:

Give yourself some credit. Those things you're doing right are not your betrayers. They're assets. They offer you an advantage over your MCI. Recognize that, and leverage them.

At the same time, we all have vulnerabilities, and MCI doesn't need much of an opening to sneak in.

Try this simple exercise. Put this book down, and get up and walk around your house, and count the number of doors and the number of windows. Come back when you're done, and write those numbers here.

Number of rooms _____

Number of windows _____

Are you back now? What did you write down? When I did this same exercise, I counted four doors and 22 windows. Are your numbers the same as mine? Probably not. We live in different houses.

Now let's imagine you're in a cold-weather climate and a polar vortex has just rolled in. The temperature outside is 5 degrees below zero. And you have left your front door wide open. That frigid air would rush into your home and chill you to the bone. You couldn't turn the furnace up high enough to make the house warm again.

What would you do? You'd slam that door shut. And then you'd wait a bit and see if the house started feeling warmer again. Hopefully it would, but what if it didn't? What if you still felt a cold draft coming from somewhere? You'd walk through the house and check the windows. Maybe one of them is open.

The defense of your cognition isn't all that different.

Exercise. Diet. Stress management. Sleep. Think of these as the four main doorways to cognition. Leave one or more of those doors open, and MCI is free to waltz in.

The tighter you shut those doors, the better protected you are. But plenty of other things still can cause cognitive impairment, or accelerate it. These are the "windows" that provide MCI with another way to come at you.

Bill is a smoker. Samantha has a vitamin D deficiency. Geraldine resides alone in a remote area and has little contact with other people. Randy drinks heavily. Gwendolyn has borderline diabetes. Hassan lives in a house with dangerously high levels of mold. Walter has hearing loss but refuses to wear his hearing aids.

Seven different people, each with his or her own unique vulnerability. Yet in each case, that window can be closed, giving them a real chance to halt or reverse their cognitive loss.

WHAT IS YOUR ACHILLES HEEL?

You're not Bill or Gwendolyn or Hassan. We're here to address you and your version of MCI.

So cognitively speaking, what is your Achilles heel? When you hone in on that and put your focus there, that's when you can really begin to turn the tables on your MCI.

Dr. Dean Sherzai, co-director of the Brain Health and Alzheimer's Prevention Program at Loma Linda University Medical Center, says this assessment of individual risk has been a difference-maker for his patients with mild cognitive impairment.

"When somebody has MCI, they have memory problems, so they come to us," he says. "At that stage, if you address their particular weaknesses and build upon their strengths, repeatedly we've seen a reversal of cognitive decline in our clinic."

But that's not done with platitudes. It's done with precision.

"We can improve your diet and your exercise and all that, but we also have to address your particular weaknesses," Dr. Sherzai says. "If you have sleep apnea and you're not addressing it, you could be eating a truck full of kale and avoid all the butter on the planet, and you still won't heal your brain. You have to address your needs."

So what do your needs look like? What is it about your unique version of MCI that makes it yours and yours alone? To determine that, you (and your doctor) will need to do some sleuthing. But here are three ways you might go about it.

OPTION NO. 1 — ASK CAPTAIN OBVIOUS

The greatest threat to your cognition may already be apparent to you. We all eat. We all sleep. And we know whether we're eating well and sleeping well. If we're not, those are risk factors that can be addressed.

If you've been sedentary, that's another major risk, and a good place for anyone with MCI to start. If your demanding boss or fast-pace life or hellish commute have you stressed to the max, and you are not addressing that stress, that's something you can't afford to ignore. (We'll take a deeper dive into stress in Chapter 10.)

But obviousness has its limitations. What's causing your MCI may not be obvious, and what's obvious may not apply in your case. You may have to plumb deeper.

OPTION NO. 2 — DO YOUR OWN RISK ASSESSMENT

There are good tools out there you can use to evaluate your brain health, identify your strengths and reveal your vulnerabilities.

One marvelous resource is the Healthy Brains tool offered by the Cleveland Clinic. You'll find it online at healthybrains.org. When you arrive on the landing page, it invites to you to take a free Brain Checkup.

Once you sign up, it walks you through a survey that takes about 10 minutes to complete. You'll answer questions about your heart health, level of exercise, diet, social engagement, sleep and mental well-being. When you're done, it gives you an overall score for your Brain Health Index, and individual scores for each of the six pillars of brain health it evaluates you for. In any area where your score looks low to you, it offers tips on how you can improve.

Another excellent option is the Team Sherzai Risk Assessment. It's available in their book *The Alzheimer's Solution,* which I consider one of the three must-reads for anyone with MCI. At the end of Chapter 2 in the Sherzai book, you'll find a seven-page Risk Assessment that you can fill out.

It looks like one of those quizzes you see in popular magazines. It asks you a set of questions and you assign a number for each answer. When you're done, the Sherzais show you how to interpret the results. In particular, you're looking to see how low or high you score in the modifiable risk factors — the things you can do something about. The higher your score, the greater the opportunity to alter the course of your cognition through some combination of medical treatment and healthier habits.

These are great tools, and I encourage you to try either or both of them. To Go Cogno is to become an advocate for your own care and the architect of your own actions. This approach lets you be both.

But depending on the complexity and persistence of your cognitive impairment, this sort of self-sleuthing may not get you all the way to an answer.

You may need to turn to the tools of precision medicine, as wielded by a medical professional who is specially trained in how they apply to MCI.

OPTION NO. 3 – GET A "COGNOSCOPY" OR SIMILAR ASSESSMENT

The concept of a "cognoscopy" is quite new to the treatment of mild cognitive impairment and Alzheimer's. It's a term coined by Dr. Dale Bredesen in his New York Times best-selling book, *The End of Alzheimer's,* and it refers to a form of highly sophisticated testing designed to pinpoint the probable causes of cognitive decline.

Dr. Bredesen is a controversial figure in the field of Alzheimer's treatment, and you are welcome to buy into his theories or not. But I will say this about his book: I consider it another of my must-reads for anyone with MCI. It is loaded with valuable information you can benefit from, regardless of the underlying cause of your cognitive impairment.

Genetics. Inflammation. Infections. Hormonal status. Toxic exposure. Gut biome. A vitamin deficiency. Body mass index. Prediabetes. Bredesen says any of these can contribute to memory loss. In fact, for someone with MCI, he suggests anywhere from 10 to 25 of such indicators may be out of whack. A cognoscopy is a set of lab tests and other exams designed to find what's gone awry.

You can get a cognoscopy from a Bredesen-trained specialist. You can undertake a cognoscopy on your own and then have a specialist interpret the results for you. You can turn to any number of MCI specialty clinics that offer their own version of this testing.

I'm not saying a cognoscopy is the right choice for. I'm saying it's an option and one you ought to be aware of. It can be pricey. But even looking into it may introduce you to a possible cause of MCI that would never have occurred to you otherwise.

And that might be helpful. If it turns out to be the culprit.

Because ultimately, you're not looking for the causes of MCI. You're looking for what triggered yours.

TIPPNG THE BALANCE

You know what irks me? When I hear a neurologist say, "You can do everything right and still get Alzheimer's."

The truth is, nobody does everything right, and that's OK. Because you don't have to. You just have to do enough to tip the cognitive balance back in your favor.

Our brain takes a beating over the course of a lifetime, even if we're being good to it, which we often aren't.

But the human brain is amazingly resilient. It absorbs all sorts of insults and injuries over many years, yet by tapping into its reserves, it compensates for them and continues to function in a cognitively normal range. Remember the old Timex watch commercials? "It takes a licking and keeps on ticking." That's your brain.

Until it takes one lick too many, and the mind begins to falter. There's an emerging theory to suggest that's what happens with MCI. Some additional hit occurs, and the accumulation of harms becomes more than the brain can compensate for. The result is cognitive impairment.

At that point, if you've caught it early enough, and if you're willing to act aggressively enough, there is still an opportunity to come to the cognitive rescue of your poor, beleaguered brain.

Not by hoping. Not by distressing. Not by guessing.

By assessing.

When you determine what your deficits are, what it was that came along and knocked your cognition out of kilter, that's when you can begin to make the changes in your life that are necessary to swing the balance back in your brain's favor.

MCI prefers to lurk in the shadows, mysterious and sinister. But as you gain a greater understanding of it, you will see that it is not the bogeyman under the bed. It is a medical condition. It has causes, and there are ways to address those causes and give yourself a legitimate shot at slowing, halting or reversing it.

The odds of someone with MCI doing that are actually pretty good and your odds only get better when you identify the strengths you have to build upon, and the vulnerabilities that leave you most susceptible to your version of MCI.

Doing some form of assessment, whether on your own or under the care of a medical pro, can help you understand what those vulnerabilities are.

MCI hopes you don't. It would rather your defenses remain down. This is your opportunity to disappoint it.

TAKEAWAYS FROM CHAPTER 4

You are the only person who has your version of MCI, and your best opportunity to slow, halt or reverse it lies in an approach that's tailored to you.

Think of exercise, diet, stress and sleep as the four main doorways to cognition. Leave one or more of those "doors" open, and MCI is free to waltz in.

Even if you slam those doors shut, there still may be an open "window" that lets MCI in, such as smoking, alcohol abuse, a vitamin deficiency, diabetes, social isolation or exposure to mold.

There are tools to help you evaluate your brain health, identify your strengths and reveal your vulnerabilities. You can do a self-assessment, or get a "cognoscopy" or similar medical analysis.

ONE ACTION, RIGHT NOW: Go to the Healthy Brains website and take their Free Brain Checkup.

CHAPTER 5 — What Is Your Why?

YOU HAVE so many questions about MCI, and this book seeks to offers answers.

But there's one question only you can answer.

What is your why?

I pose that question now, because a journey like the one you're about to embark on has a greater chance of success when driven by a why — a purpose, a reason to do the things that will be asked of you.

A sense of purpose (what the Japanese call *ikigai*) is one of our more powerful protections against cognitive impairment.

Sure, other things help, too. Exercise. Diet. Sleep. Stress reduction. Brain training. We'll get to all of these and more in the chapters ahead.

But don't underestimate the power of purpose.

When you bring a deeply personal and compelling "why" to health behavior change, you are more likely to sustain the effort and more likely to succeed.

In fact, a sense of purpose can be a form of cognitive therapy all by itself.

In a study published in the *Archives of General Psychiatry*, researchers followed nearly a thousand older adults. Over the next seven years, about one in six ended up with dementia.

But those who expressed the greatest sense of purpose in life at the beginning of the study were the least likely to develop Alzheimer's disease. They also had the lowest rates of MCI.

Eric Kim, a research fellow at Harvard's T.H. Chan School of Public Health, says even people with emerging signs of Alzheimer's are more able to sustain their cognition and quality of life when driven by a sense of purpose.

"Even when people have the same amount of biological markers in the brain, those who have a higher sense of purpose can actually function better," Kim told me. "They are somehow pushing themselves to continue functioning, even though they are biologically having the same amount of tangles in their brain."

So how about you? What would give purpose to your efforts?

Don't answer right away. Take time to really reflect on that.

Think about what it is you are trying to accomplish, and what it would mean in your life if you were able to achieve it.

What if you were to reverse your MCI? What if you could stop it where it is now, and not get any worse? Or slow it down, and extend the quality of your life and the time you have with loved ones?

What would that mean in your life? What would you do with that gift?

Maybe it's that trip to Paris you've always dreamed of. Or the book you've been meaning to write. Or that yearning to learn how to paint or play the piano.

It doesn't have to be some grand ambition. It just has to be meaningful to you, like getting together once a year with old college friends or volunteering at your granddaughter's elementary school.

Identify that why. Picture it in your mind. And then write it down. On paper. And put it in a place where you will see it every day.

Let it be a constant reminder of what you're working toward, and why your cognition is worth defending.

MCI isn't overcome by accident. It's something that's done on purpose. And better yet, with a sense of purpose. What's yours?

ONE ACTION, RIGHT NOW: Write down your "why" and put it where you'll see it every day.

CHAPTER 6 — A Call To Action

MCI IS A LOT of things, but most of all, it's a bully.

It wants to puff out its chest. It wants to bare its teeth. It wants to leave you feeling like you have no chance at all.

So let me assure you otherwise. It is absolutely possible to slow, halt or reverse mild cognitive impairment. In fact, it's more than possible. It's likely.

These days, experts can tell us with confidence that over a period of four or five years, most people with MCI will see their cognitive loss stabilize or get better.

Let's look at hard numbers.

Researchers at the University of Pittsburgh followed nearly 900 adults with mild cognitive impairment over a period of five years, to see how they fared.

The results, published in the *Journal of the American Geriatrics Society*, showed that

- 53 percent stabilized at MCI,
- 35 percent reverted to cognitively normal or fluctuated between MCI and normal cognition, and
- only 12 percent progressed to dementia.

The findings caught many neurologists by surprise. They've spent their career describing MCI as a "precursor" to dementia, or as an "intermediate step leading to Alzheimer's." And they've blithely passed that sense of hopelessness on to their patients.

So let's correct that notion right now. You shouldn't assume that a diagnosis of MCI dooms you to dementia, and doctors shouldn't either.

I have that from the best possible source — Dr. Mary Ganguli, a geriatric psychiatrist who led the research study in Pittsburgh. Having seen what actually happened across a large, general population of people with MCI, she's ready to retire the misperception that MCI invariably leads to dementia.

"We want people to understand that not all mild cognitive impairment is MCI due to Alzheimer's, and I think it's come to mean that," Dr. Ganguli told me. "In general parlance, people have come to think MCI is the stage before dementia and it isn't."

Doctors need to hear that message, but people with MCI need to hear it even more.

Because it offers hope. It gives you a reason to try.

Although I want you to understand that this book has a clear intent, and it's not to help you try. It's to help you succeed.

"ROUND UP THE USUAL SUSPECTS"

I am never surprised when someone with MCI is able to halt or reverse their cognitive decline. I see it all the time. Some do it with the help of a really good doctor. Some figure it out almost entirely on their own.

Usually, medication plays only a minor role. This is something that's done more by will than by pill.

It's done by people who are determined to defend their cognition and willing to make changes in their life that have been scientifically shown to stabilize or improve cognition and prevent dementia.

They began by heeding the call of Captain Renault from that classic scene at the end of *Casablanca*, when he says: "Round up the usual suspects."

Exercise. Diet. Stress reduction. Restorative sleep. Brain training. These are where the experts suggest you start, and the research tells us how right they are. Invariably, the people whom I've seen put their emphasis in these areas are the ones who ended up getting results.

How well these work for you will depend on where you're starting from. But all by themselves, they may be enough to halt or reverse your cognitive loss. And what if they did? Wouldn't that be great?

Well, then let's Go Cogno and make that happen for you. All of us are capable of greatness, once we understand how unassumingly it can be achieved. If there is a call to action I can offer you, let it be this quote from Thomas Fowell Buxton, who said:

"With ordinary talent and extraordinary perseverance, all things are attainable."

When I look at the people whom I have seen halt or reverse their MCI, not one of them reached into the sky and brought down a lightning bolt. There is not one single thing they did that I would describe as bold or dramatic.

They are just ordinary, everyday people who said, "Dammit, I want my mind back. My cognition is worth defending, and I'm going to defend it." And they set about making small, simple changes in their life and sustained the effort long enough to let those things work for them.

There is nothing at all magnificent about what they did — except the result. And what they achieved is every bit as available to you.

Yes, you will have to put in the work, just as they did. But the changes you need to make in your life can be broken down into tiny actions that are well within your capability.

Especially now that MCI has given you a wonderful weapon to use against it.

RIDING THE MOTIVATION WAVE

Even as you begin, you already have a huge advantage.

One of the biggest reasons people fail to make lifestyle changes is because they aren't sufficiently motivated. They're comfortably nestled in their current habits, and that sense of complacency is greater than whatever half-hearted intention they have to live in a healthier way. They know they ought to get some exercise. And when are they going to do that? Eh, maybe tomorrow. Today they'd rather sit on the couch, binge-watching *Game of Thrones* and eating a bag of chips.

Most people with MCI don't have that problem. They are highly motivated to make changes. What's going wrong in their brain frightens the crap out of them. They're desperate to do something about it.

BJ Fogg, a psychologist and director of the Persuasive Technology Lab at Stanford, says one of the surest ways to make a healthy habit stick is by tapping your motivation when you feel it most. He says:

> *"Motivation only has one role in our lives and that's to help us to do hard things."*

In the average person, the level of motivation ebbs and flows. For them, Fogg says it's about taking action at that moment when they feel unusually inspired to make a change. He calls it riding the "motivation wave."

For people with MCI, their diagnosis provides the ultimate motivation wave. It's more like a tsunami. When you catch a wave that big, you have all the impetus you need to succeed.

Then it just becomes a matter of choosing where to channel your efforts.

This is where I see so many people with MCI get stuck. They've got a barrage of confusing, conflicting information coming at them, and it leaves them bewildered. Either it paralyzes them, so they do nothing at all, or they end up grasping at the latest thing someone shared on Facebook, hoping against hope that it will somehow do them some good.

Let's cut through the chaos and put you on a clear, proven course of action that has helped so many others before you halt or reverse their MCI.

MEDICATION NATION, BUT NOT FOR MCI

It starts with the right mindset.

Mild cognitive impairment can be a frightening, devastating diagnosis. So many questions race through your head. "Can I stop it? Can it be reversed?" Fortunately, you now have those answers.

Often, the next question becomes, "OK, then, what can I take for it?"

That is what traditional medicine has taught us to want. You go to the doctor, and the doctor gives you a pill. Americans have been conditioned to pop pills in their mouth in a way that reminds me of Lucy and Ethel in the chocolate factory. Some 4.3 billion prescriptions are written in the United States every year, and we spend an estimated $200 billion annually on medications that are unnecessary or improper.

With MCI, it's not so much about unnecessary prescriptions. It's that the doctor doesn't have a pill to give you in the first place.

There is no FDA-approved medication for mild cognitive impairment.

There are a handful of "off-label" medicines that may help a little, so your doctor might suggest one of them. And there are some medical conditions that can cause or contribute to MCI (for example, hypertension or hyperthyroidism), and you might get medication for that.

But for many people with cognitive impairment, medication won't be in the mix. Some of the top MCI doctors tell me that when they see a new patient, they are more likely to start weaning that person off some of the medications they're already on than to prescribe more.

And even if you go to one of the elite cognitive clinics — the kind that provide individualized, precision care for MCI — and say, "My brain isn't working right, give me something for it," among the first things they're likely to give you are a fitness coach and a nutritionist.

So please understand that going in. Mild cognitive impairment is a complex, chronic, lifestyle-related condition, and the answers to it are primarily found in what the experts call "modifiable risk factors."

In other words, health behaviors.

That's where the opportunity is. Want proof? Here's just a sampling of recent scientific evidence.

EXERCISE

The study: Sixty people age 60 or older, all with MCI. Half did aerobic exercise for 12 months. The other half served as the control group.

The result: The people with MCI who exercised regularly showed a 47 percent improvement in memory scores.

DIET

The study: More than 900 people between the ages of 58 and 98 were tracked for several years. Half were put on the MIND Diet, a nutrition plan designed to benefit cognition.

The result: Those who rigorously followed the MIND diet reduced their risk for Alzheimer's by 53 percent.

STRESS MANAGEMENT

The study: Sixty people who scored in the range of MCI. To lower stress, they spent 12 minutes a day listening to relaxing classical music or meditating.

The result: At the end of six months, they were tested again, and their memory had improved so much that, on average, they'd returned to cognitively normal.

RESTORATIVE SLEEP

The study: Some 2,500 people between the ages of 55 and 90, whose medical histories were studied over many years to see what role sleep played in their risk of cognitive impairment.

The result: Among those who had sleep apnea or some other sleep disorder, the average age they developed MCI was 77. Those with no sleep disorder did not experience MCI until an average age of 90.

BRAIN TRAINING

The study: Some 120 people over the age of 65 who were diagnosed with MCI or reported subjective cognitive decline. Those in the intervention group met with a dietician and an exercise physiologist to set up individual plans, and also used the BrainHQ app for brain training.

The result: Those in the intervention group showed a significant improvement in cognitive function and a significant decline in Alzheimer's risk.

In the world of medical research, these are incredible results. If a medicine came along that could deliver results like these, it would be declared a "blockbuster" drug, and the scientists who discovered it would be lining up to collect their Nobel Prizes.

Someday, we will have miracle drugs for MCI and dementia. But you don't have to wait for that. You can get these results right now.

Just by doing the what participants in these studies did. By choosing to defend your cognition and then channeling your efforts into the five brain health essentials that rigorous research has already ordained.

Exercise. Diet. Stress management. Restorative sleep. Brain training. Each and every one of these represents a proven way to slow, halt or reverse mild cognitive impairment all by itself. When you combine them, they become even more powerful.

The results tell us that. But even more than the results, I want you to think about the people who achieved them.

These studies weren't done with test tubes. They weren't done on mice. These studies were done on real people with MCI. They were people just like you, with all the same fears and apprehensions and dread that you have. But they were willing to put their trust and effort into making changes in their life, and it paid off for them.

What they did, you can do, too. They did it for the sake of science. Now you get to do it for the sake of your own cognition.

To introduce you to the art of the possible, I want to share with you the journey of Miriam, who started from a place of despair and over a period of more than four years, doggedly marched her way back to cognitively normal.

She didn't approach this quest exactly the way you will, but her journey can inform and inspire you as you prepare for your own. In the next chapter, I will lay out Miriam's story, to help you see what it means to Go Cogno — and how it changed her life.

TAKEAWAYS FROM CHAPTER 6

Over a period of four or five years, nearly 90 percent of people with MCI will see their cognitive loss stabilize or get better, research shows.

There is no FDA-approved drug for MCI. Instead, experts encourage you to put your efforts into these five brain health essentials: exercise, diet, stress reduction, restorative sleep and brain training.

This will require you to make changes in your life, but these changes can be broken down into tiny actions that are well within your capability, especially when you ride the "motivation wave."

ONE ACTION, RIGHT NOW: For the next week, set aside 12 minutes every day to listen to relaxing music.

CHAPTER 7 — Meet Miriam

MIRIAM REMEMBERS vividly the day she received her diagnosis — mild cognitive impairment due to vascular disease and depression. It wasn't news she was ready to hear.

"Even though I thought something was wrong, I had hoped it wasn't that bad," Miriam says. "I hoped it was just me being too worried. I guess I was a little shocked, even though I wasn't completely shocked."

Based on her family history, Miriam knew all about Alzheimer's. But mild cognitive impairment? She'd never heard of it. "I had no clue what MCI is," she says.

As for the reality of living with MCI, it hit her like she'd stepped in front of a bus.

"I was tired. I was fatigued," she says. "I tried to exercise but it felt like there was a weight on me. I couldn't focus properly. I couldn't think properly. I was scared. I had to write everything down, because I couldn't remember. I could not come home and cook dinner. I would come home and sit and watch TV. At that particular point, it was strictly that I wasn't able to thrive."

At the time she was diagnosed, Miriam was 50 years old and working as an accountant at a high-tech start-up. The company was struggling. Her manager got laid off. Soon after, they laid her off, too.

"During the time when I was let go, I was feeling so much anxiety," Miriam says. "I decided I didn't want to start another job yet. I wanted to get some of this anxiety down."

She wasn't sure where to turn or what to do. But one idea did occur to her. Maybe she'd have a better shot if she were under the care of a top-notch neurologist who really understood her condition.

"I started searching to see if I could find a doctor, someone who I could trust, who knew something about dementia," she says.

"I knew there really was no cure, but I thought if I could find someone who was really into it, they would be on the front line and be aware of something if it did come up."

That was the first big turning point for Miriam.

To Go Cogno is to be an advocate for your own care and the architect of your own actions. Two of the most fundamental ways you do that are by

- having a diagnosis you understand and can act on, and
- finding the right doctor.

Miriam had done both. She had her diagnosis. She had a good memory specialist. She was ready to get to work.

EXERCISE AND DIET AS A START

By then, Miriam had come to understand that even if there's no medicine approved for the treatment of MCI, there's an abundance of evidence that lifestyle changes can halt or reverse it.

She took up an exercise program, coupled with dramatic changes to her diet.

"I started walking with my husband," Miriam says. "We would walk three times during the week, three or four miles. On weekend days, we'd walk four to eight miles each day. It was hard. I felt like I had weights on my legs."

But she persevered. Those regular walks turned into a healthy habit she continues today, and that fatigue has been replaced by a feeling of vigor. "I still do about that much walking, but I walk a lot faster now," she says. "I'm not dragging. I have pep. I have energy. I feel a lot younger."

For Miriam, a bigger turning point came when a physician assistant who worked for her memory specialist recommended a primarily plant-based diet, with no meat, but fish two or three times a week.

She gave Miriam the book *The Perfect Gene Diet*, by Pamela McDonald, and told her to follow the eating plan recommended for people with the ApoE4 gene. That gene is associated with a higher risk of Alzheimer's.

At the time, Miriam was on several medications, including an antidepressant. Her diagnosis was MCI due to vascular disease and depression, so if she hoped to restore her cognition, she had to deal with her depression.

In the weeks after Miriam began following this new diet, she saw an unexpected benefit. Her depressive symptoms began to ease. She never wanted to be on that medication in the first place, because of the side effects. Soon, she stopped needing it at all.

"Four months after being on The Perfect Gene Diet — and I followed it strictly — I was no longer on an anti-depressant," Miriam says. "The diet cleared up my depression, so I continued doing the diet. I followed the diet, except no meat whatsoever. I only did fish."

(Please note, there is some evidence that changes in diet can help reduce the symptoms of depression and Miriam got a better result than most, but there is no proven dietary cure for depression.)

SEARCHING FOR THE RIGHT CLUES

The brisk walks and the changes in diet were making a difference for Miriam, although she had a ways to go yet.

"I felt a little bit better, my mind was a little clearer," she says. "But I was still having trouble."

And from then on, it became more of a detective story. She and her doctors were looking for clues. How could she make more progress? What did her brain need that it still wasn't getting?

One of the earliest clues had been what it didn't need: red meat.

Most of us can eat a brain-healthy diet and still enjoy a steak or a burger every now and then. The Mediterranean diet and the MIND diet both allow limited amounts of red meat. So did the diet Miriam was following.

But that turned out to be the wrong choice for Miriam. She was working with a physician's assistant to improve her diet. "She told me, 'Your body doesn't process meat very well,'" Miriam says. "She recommended I go plant-based but eat fish two or three times a week."

Later on, Miriam would shift entirely to a whole-food, plant-based (WFPB) diet. She hoped it would lower her cholesterol level, which was dangerously high and required her to be on medication.

In some people, eating a WFPB diet can lower LDL (bad) cholesterol. That's what Miriam was hoping for. She wanted to get off statins and be medicine free.

But that didn't happen for her. Despite her efforts to eat better, her cholesterol level barely budged. It felt like such a defeat.

But some people have a hereditary risk for high cholesterol, which leaves them genetically unable to lower their cholesterol through diet alone. No matter how well they eat, cholesterol continues to build up in their bloodstream. For them, medication may be necessary.

So Miriam stayed on statins and learned a valuable lesson. This MCI she had was an individualized thing. It's good to know what works for other people, but she had to find what worked for her.

"Each of us is different," she says. "We have to work within our own situation to find solutions."

"MOVING FORWARD AND GETTING WELL"

Miriam was doing better — well enough, in fact, to return to the workforce.

But going back to work was a mixed blessing. With her new job came a whole new shockwave of work-related stress.

"I didn't feel comfortable working; I was scared," she says. "I had to write everything down, because I was afraid at work I would forget something. I didn't want to meet with people and talk about something I did because I couldn't remember things."

If she was going to reclaim her cognition, she had to deal with both her stress and the emotional toll MCI was taking on her.

"Around mid-2016, I started going to a therapist," she says. "I did individual therapy for two and a half years, and I also did about a year of group therapy. That helped me in this whole process of growing and changing things in my life, and moving forward and getting well."

She also learned some stress-reduction strategies and began to use them regularly.

One was a visualization technique that taught her how to leave her stress at work. "I was bringing things home from work mentally," she says. "So I would visualize putting whatever that concern was in a jar, putting the lid on the jar and setting that jar on the desk at my office before I left work."

She used a simple breathing technique as well. "Breathe in, breathe out slowly," she says. "Letting go, just relaxing."

THE STORY THAT MATTERS IS YOURS

It was all adding up for Miriam. With each change she made in her life, with each vulnerability she addressed, she drew closer to her goal. She had halted her MCI and was on the verge of reversing it.

Remember what we learned earlier in the book. It's not about being perfect. You don't have to do everything right. You just have to do enough to tip the cognitive balance back in your brain's favor.

That's what Miriam was doing, and that's what I have seen so many other people with MCI do.

If I shared six of their stories, or 16 of their stories, you would see the same recurring themes. It's better to have a definitive diagnosis, but some didn't. It helps to have a top-notch doc, but again, some didn't. Yet their stories always seem to converge around the things they did. They got their body moving, they nourished their brain, and they tamped down their stress.

Some had other vulnerabilities to tend to. Later in this book, you will meet Per Laursen, who would never have overcome MCI without addressing his sleep apnea. You'll also meet Steve Raymond, who went all-in on exercise and diet but got the greatest cognitive boost when he discovered brain training. I could tell you the stories of so many others just like them.

But the only story that matters is yours.

I'm not here to dwell on the experiences of others. Nor am I here to fill your heads with facts. Most of the people whom I've been introducing you to started out with far less knowledge that you will gain by reading this book. But knowledge wasn't what saved them.

The truest thing about the people I have seen halt or reverse their MCI is that they didn't knowledge their way there. They did their way there. I'm here to help you be a doer.

I don't want to be the three-hundredth person to tell you, "Eat blueberries." I want to be the person who convinces you to take one action to defend your cognition. And then another action. And then another.

That's how I have seen people halt or reverse their MCI. By playing the long game. Tiny, tiny changes. One little thing they were ready to do. Followed by the next.

How long did they keep that up? As long as it took.

Early on, when the results weren't obvious, something kept them going. I can't say what it was. Hope? Faith? Orneriness? An inner strength that even they didn't know they possessed? Maybe all of the above.

But they stuck with it long enough for the little things they were doing to become habits, and for those habits to become powerful.

I am a big believer in affirmations. We should all take a moment every day to affirm ourselves.

This morning, on the day I am writing these words to you, my affirmation was a quote from Anne Frank. She said:

> "How wonderful it is that nobody need wait a single moment before starting to improve the world."

In that spirit, let me paraphrase this wise child.

How wonderful it is that nobody need wait a single moment before beginning to defend their cognition.

The time to Go Cogno is now.

TAKEAWAYS FROM CHAPTER 7

When acting in defense of your cognition, unless exercise and diet are already a strength for you, those are two good places to start.

MCI requires an individualized approach. It's good to know what works for other people, but you need to find what works for you.

The people whom I have seen halt or reverse their MCI didn't knowledge their way there. They did their way there. Be a do-er.

How wonderful it is that you need not wait a single moment before beginning to defend your cognition.

ONE ACTION, RIGHT NOW: Review Miriam's story and write down one thing she did that you're inspired by and feel ready to do.

CHAPTER 8 - Get Your Body Moving

ALZHEIMER'S IS what we all fear. No one wants Alzheimer's. And there are a handful of places on the planet where virtually no one gets it.

You may have heard of these rare locales. They're known as the "Blue Zones," and there are only five of them in the world.

These far-flung places — from Sarnia, Italy, to Okinawa, Japan, to Loma Linda, California — couldn't be more different geographically or ethnically. But here's what they have in common: They share a set of lifestyle characteristics that leave their inhabitants all but immune to chronic health problems like heart disease, stroke and yes, even Alzheimer's. Their brains simply aren't susceptible to it.

The Blue Zones are close-knit communities, where people share deep family bonds and strong social connections. They are religious people, whose faith gives them purpose. But it's more than that. There are two things in particular that keep them mentally sharp, even into their 80s or 90s.

First, they don't live life in a seated position. They stay physically active. And second, when they do sit down to eat, they heap their plates with brain-friendly food.

Exercise and diet. That's what helps keep them cognitively intact.

Granted, you don't live in a Blue Zone and you aren't likely to pack up and move to Nicoya, Costa Rica, or the Greek island of Ikaria anytime soon.

Fortunately, you don't have to. You just have to eat like an Ikarian. And exercise like one.

So let's get your body moving.

THE "WONDER DRUG" KNOWN AS EXERCISE

For mild cognitive impairment and many other medical maladies, exercise is the closest thing we have to a miracle. That's according to the Academy of Medical Royal Colleges, which issued a landmark 2015 report titled "Exercise — The Miracle Cure."

I don't expect you to read this 59-page report, but do yourself a favor and check out this breezy 5-minute video by Dr. Mike Evans. It's a fun, engaging tribute to the awesomeness of exercise as a treatment for MCI or any other chronic disease you can think of. This video will help you understand why Sue Bailey, chair of the Academy of Medical Royal Colleges, says: "If physical activity was a drug, it would be classified as a wonder drug."

Indeed, exercise can be as good as or better than medicine in every way but one. It doesn't come in a pill. It's not something you take; it's something you do. But if you're willing to do it, the cognitive benefits are clear. Here's just one example.

You know what Miracle-Gro is, right? You sprinkle some on a plant, and it grows like crazy.

Wouldn't it be nice if there were something like that for your brain? Actually, there is.

It's called brain-derived neurotrophic factor, or BDNF for short. Harvard professor Dr. John Ratey gave it the nickname "Miracle-Gro for the brain" because when scientists put BDNF on nerve cells, they could literally see the cells begin to grow.

One recent study found older adults with the highest levels of BDNF had a 50 percent slower loss of memory and thinking skills than those with the lowest levels.

Getting your body moving also increases blood flow to the brain, which can benefit cognition. In a recent study, scientists mapped changes in the brain that occurred in older adults who did aerobic exercise for one year. They saw improved blood flow in regions of the brain important to memory. Even the older adults with memory issues saw improved cognition as a result.

If you're serious about slowing, halting or reversing cognitive decline, you will not find a clearer consensus than the one around exercise. It's the single best suggestion anyone can offer you, and it's the single best action you can take on behalf of your brain.

To help you get started, here are answers to some of the most frequent questions people with MCI have about physical activity.

WHAT IS THE BEST EXERCISE FOR MCI?

There is not one form of exercise that's been shown to be better than another. That's good news, because it allows you to choose. So pick a style of exercise you enjoy; you'll be more likely to stick with it.

For cognition, aerobic exercise seems particularly beneficial. That would be any activity that moderately raises your heart rate and causes you to break a sweat. The rule of thumb is, if you can talk but not sing while doing an activity, it's moderately aerobic.

For many people with MCI, a brisk walk becomes the exercise of choice. It's something they can do in their neighborhood or at a park, or at a rec center or a shopping mall, for that matter. Walking in nature has been shown to offer an additional cognitive benefit.

Other gentle, accessible forms of physical activity for people who have been sedentary are water aerobics or tai chi. A recent study found that for people with MCI, engaging in tai chi can "significantly improve global cognitive function, memory and learning."

For a more balanced exercise program, you can also include strength training and exercises that improve balance and flexibility. Another emerging trend is special cross-fit training for older adults with chronic conditions. But don't feel like you have to transform yourself into a gym warrior. The important thing is to get your body moving.

HOW MUCH EXERCISE DO I NEED TO DO?

The World Health Organization recently issued a major report on exercise as a way to prevent dementia and cognitive decline. It recommends:

- Older adults should do at least 150 minutes a week of moderate-intensity aerobic activity, or 75 minutes a week of vigorous-intensity aerobics.
- For an optimal benefit, over time you can increase that to 300 minutes a week of moderate-intensity aerobic activity, or 150 minutes a week of vigorous-intensity aerobics.
- Bouts of aerobic activity should last at least 10 minutes.
- If you have poor mobility, you are encouraged to do balance exercises at least three times a week.
- Muscle-strengthening exercises are also encouraged twice a week or more.

HOW LONG WILL IT TAKE TO START SEEING RESULTS?

Exercise is not a quick fix, cognitively speaking. The benefits can be great, but it takes time for them to materialize. Studies have shown you need to engage in regular physical activity for six months to a year before you can expect to see measurable changes in cognition.

This is a lifestyle change you want to make and sustain. You want to define yourself as a person who is physically active and incorporate that into your life on an ongoing basis.

I HATE GOING TO THE GYM. DO I HAVE TO?

No, the only thing you have to do is find the form of physical activity that's right for you and engage in it on a regular basis.

When you study the Blue Zones, where MCI and dementia are nearly nonexistent, there is no exercise culture. They don't hit the gym. They live in physically active ways that keep their body moving without having to schedule weekly workouts. That includes walking, gardening and the kinds of physical labor and chores that have been replaced by machines or electronics in the Western world.

Vacuuming the floor or mowing the lawn or raking leaves are forms of moderately aerobic physical activity. If that's not your thing, how about ballroom dancing? In one study, involving 60 people with MCI, those who engaged in a form of aerobic dancing showed improvement in cognitive function, especially memory and brain processing speed.

Other choices include rowing, golf, walking the dog or Zumba, to suggest just a few.

Even if you have physical limitations, there are still good options for you these days. Chair yoga is becoming increasingly popular. Getting a good workout in on a recumbent bike is an option, too.

I'd also encourage you to check the availability of a chair-based program called "Ageless Grace," which is specifically designed to combine physical activity with cognitive challenges that can improve brain function.

START SLOW AND WORK YOUR WAY UP

I am obligated to issue this standard reminder. If you have not been physically active, always consult with your doctor before beginning an exercise program.

Start small, and gradually increase the intensity of your workouts. Your first goal might be to walk to the corner and back, or once around the block, and then you can build from there. Do what you feel ready to do, and let your body tell you when it's ready to take on more.

As you commit to physical activity and make it a regular part of your life, you'll discover that the benefits aren't just cognitive. You'll feel more energy. You'll feel less stressed. Your mood will improve.

So will your appetite. Which means it's time to become more intentional about how you feed your brain and body. That's what we'll talk about next.

TAKEAWAYS FROM CHAPTER 8

For mild cognitive impairment and many other medical maladies, exercise is the closest thing we have to a miracle. The Academy of Medical Royal Colleges calls it a "wonder drug."

There is not one form of exercise that's been shown to be better than another. Pick a style of exercise you enjoy; you'll be more likely to stick with it.

Older adults should shoot for at least 150 minutes a week of moderate-intensity aerobic activity, or 75 minutes a week of vigorous-intensity aerobics.

Studies have shown you need to engage in regular physical activity for six months to a year before you can expect to see measurable changes in cognition. This is a lifestyle change you want to make and sustain.

If you have not been physically active, always consult with your doctor before beginning an exercise program. Start modestly, and gradually increase the intensity of your workouts.

ONE ACTION, RIGHT NOW: Watch the fun, breezy video by Dr. Mike Evans on "the single best thing you can do for your health — exercise!" It's available here — gocogno.com/evans

CHAPTER 9 – Food For Thought

JUST AS you can exercise your way to better brain health, you can eat you can eat your way there, too.

That's not merely a good idea. It's an imperative.

As Dr. Ayesha Sherzai says, "Whatever you eat will either break the brain or make the brain."

And let's not sugarcoat this. The traditional Western diet wants to break your brain.

The way most Americans eat is fundamentally flawed in two ways, and either is enough to do serious harm. Taken together, they become a cognitive wrecking crew.

On the one hand, certain nutrients our brain need to function well are largely missing from the foods we favor.

Take omega-3s, the "good fat" that promotes brain health. Omega-3 fatty acids play the role of a cognitive lubricant. Think of them as "motor oil for the mind."

The main sources of omega-3s — things like cold-water fish, walnuts and flaxseed — are largely missing from the Western diet, and as a result, most older adults are woefully deficient in omega-3s.

I've seen estimates that 70 percent of Americans don't get enough omega-3 fatty acids, and that 20 percent have no detectable amount of omega-3s in their body at all. How well would your car run if there were no trace of motor oil in the engine?

In the Western diet, many other brain-healthy foods are missing in action as well, robbing the mind of essential nutrients. It's no wonder that the United States has the second-highest rate of Alzheimer's in the world, given the way we eat.

As the American diet has gone global, changing the eating habits of nations where dementia used to be less common, those countries are seeing their dementia rates skyrocket. We are essentially exporting Alzheimer's to the world, one cheeseburger at a time.

Because that's the other side of our eating problem. It's not just what's missing from our diet. It's also what we eat way too much of. Fast food. Fried food. Processed food. Additives. Preservatives. Refined sugar.

We love these things, but they plunder our cognition.

And yet, for all the terrible things they can do to your brain, you don't have to give them up (unless you want to). You can still eat the naughty foods you have a taste for, but you need to eat them less frequently and find ways over time to introduce some healthier choices into your diet.

That is a lesson I learned from Dr. Nate Bergman, who serves as chief scientific wellness officer at Kemper Cognitive Wellness in Cleveland and hosts the *Evolving Past Alzheimer's* podcast.

His practice focuses heavily on people with mild cognitive impairment and he insists that MCI and other neurological conditions are "generally treatable and reversible."

Dr. Bergman told me it's not about having the perfect diet. He says the big gains come when someone who has lousy eating habits makes an effort to eat better.

"Going from a poor diet to a good diet is where we see the biggest improvement," he says. "Going from a good diet to a great diet does not always equate to the same level of improvement."

A DIET THAT'S BRAIN-HEALTHY AND PROVEN TO WORK

Paleo. Keto. Gluten free. Whole foods, Plant-based. Vegan. Healthy diets are getting more attention these days, and there are so many choices now. Perhaps too many. Which one do you choose? Where do you even begin?

I encourage you to look for an eating plan that

- is specifically associated with brain health and improved cognition, and
- is backed by strong evidence showing it can help prevent, stabilize or reverse cognitive decline.

Two diets in particular meet that test.

The first is the Mediterranean Diet, a traditional way of eating in countries that border the Mediterranean Ocean. It emphasizes seafood, small portions of lean meat, fruit, vegetables, nuts, grains, olive oil and red wine.

The second is the MIND Diet, which takes the best elements of the Mediterranean Diet and a heart-healthy diet called the DASH Diet, and combines them in a way that's more intentionally designed to promote better cognition.

Dr. Bergman recommends the MIND diet, which can be an ideal choice for anyone who is looking to eat in a brain-healthy way. The MIND diet is flexible and easy to follow. It hones in on 10 foods that can help cognition and five foods that hammer cognition, and shows you how much of each to eat. And it gets results.

A study funded by the National Institute on Aging found that following the MIND diet rigorously can slash the risk of dementia by 53 percent, and even people who only follow the diet casually can lower their risk by 35 percent.

It is evidence like that, not to mention their own firsthand experience, that has convinced Drs. Dean and Ayesha Sherzai how possible it is to undo MCI.

"Absolutely you can reverse this at the MCI stage; in our own clinic, we see this on a daily basis," says Dr. Dean Sherzai, who co-directs the Brain Health and Alzheimer's prevention program at Loma Linda University Health, along with his wife, Ayesha.

For more than a decade now, the Sherzais have focused their practice on people with mild cognitive impairment. "We really think that population is most amenable to reversing," Dean Sherzai says. "And of course, the earlier you get somebody, the more likely that you will stop it."

Each of their patients gets an individualized treatment plan, but proper nutrition is central to their approach. Dean Sherzai says the right changes in diet can make all the difference. "Just nutrition alone has been shown to reverse the disease," he says.

THE "MAKE YOUR BRAIN" HEALTHY EATING CHALLENGE

You may have already gotten that message.

Many people with MCI know how important diet and nutrition are to cognitive well-being. They know they should be eating in a healthier way and they want to make changes. They just need a little help in deciding what changes to make and how to turn those changes into healthy habits that last.

That's what led to me to develop the "Make Your Brain" Healthy Eating Challenge, which I'm offering to you in combination with this book.

This simple challenge will help you improve your diet in ways that make your brain healthier, more resilient, and better able to fend off MCI.

The challenge is free and designed for someone who knows they're not eating right, and really wants to make some changes.

If you are determined to Go Cogno and defend your cognition, the "Make Your Brain" Healthy Eating Challenge is an ideal way to get started. When you join the challenge, here's what you'll get out of it:

- You'll learn what foods can "Make Your Brain" and what foods can "Break Your Brain."
- You'll identify easy ways to improve your diet and better nourish your brain.
- You'll get the tools you need to make those changes and turn them into lasting habits.
- And you'll walk away with the confidence and momentum to keep right on refining your diet in brain-healthy ways, giving yourself a better chance of halting or reversing cognitive decline.

I'm offering an invitation for you to join this Healthy Eating Challenge right now, and you'll get an invitation again at the end of the book.

Either way, I hope you step up to the challenge. It's a chance to change your eating habits for good.

TAKEAWAYS FROM CHAPTER 9

The way you eat can either "break the brain" or "make the brain."

The traditional Western diet lacks the nutrients your brain needs to function well, and it's overloaded with things we know harm cogni-

tion, including fast food, fried food, processed food, preservatives, and refined sugar.

Choose a diet that's specifically associated with brain health and backed by science. Both the Mediterranean Diet and the MIND Diet meet that test.

The MIND diet is flexible and easy to follow. It hones in on 10 foods that can help cognition and five foods that hammer cognition, and shows you how much of each to eat.

ONE ACTION, RIGHT NOW: Sign up for the "Make Your Brain" Healthy Eating Challenge at: gocogno.com/myb-challenge

CHAPTER 10 – Address Your Stress

IF THERE were a "Public Enemy" list for mild cognitive impairment, stress would be right up near the top. Stress is the John Dillinger, the Ma Barker, the Baby Face Nelson of cognition. Prolonged, unaddressed stress can brutalize your brain.

One neurologist I know has a vivid way of describing the cognitive impact of stress. He calls it "a sledgehammer to the head."

Research confirms his warning. Consider that

- a study done at the Albert Einstein College of Medicine found older adults with high levels of chronic stress are twice as likely to develop MCI, and
- in another study involving people already diagnosed with MCI, those with higher levels of stress saw faster cognitive decline.

Even if you didn't feel wildly stressed out in your previous life, now that you've been diagnosed with MCI, you may find that stress has gotten its claws into you. It's essential that you learn to deal with it.

Not all stress is bad stress. There are types of short-term stress that can be good for us. Maybe you've been asked to speak in public and the idea terrifies you. But you pull it off and present yourself well. Once the speech is over, the stress dissipates.

The wrong kind of stress is the unrelenting kind. It goes on and on.

It's not driven by some positive goal or some challenge you've willingly undertaken.

It's the kind of stress you felt when you were in third grade and you went to school every day knowing that bully was waiting for you. It's the stress of a job where you put in 10-hour days and still end up bringing work home with you. It's the stress of feeling like a slave to your cell phone and the ping of every new email or text message that demands your attention.

When you're under stress, your brain triggers a natural alarm system in your body. In the short term, it puts you in a heightened state of readiness to deal with whatever you're facing. But when the stress goes on and on, the alarm system doesn't shut off. It keeps pumping hormones that eventually become corrosive in ways that do damage to your stomach, your heart and your cognition.

That kind of stress will not let go of you. You have to learn to let go of it.

How might you do that? The way you have in the past, when you weren't even trying to (or maybe you were).

LIFE IS A BEACH

Let's compare vacation stories. I'll tell you mine, then you reflect on yours.

My wife has family in northern California, so we try to vacation out there when we can. There's a place we usually stay. A short walk down a sandy path leads us to the ocean. It's not a sunbathing beach. It's more natural and rugged. Most days, there's hardly anyone there. Maybe a guy in a hooded sweatshirt and shorts letting his dog run loose. A woman jogging barefoot. A few surfers, if the waves are good.

We walk down to the outdoor pool, swim a few laps, and stroll back, soothed by the distinct smell of salt water and the sound of the lapping waves. Often, when we start back, it's still foggy. But by the time we get home, pour that first cup of coffee and settle into a chair on the deck, the mist has lifted and the sun peeks over the eastern hills, warming our faces and feet.

At that moment, not a care in the world can reach me. I can't help but think, "Man, if this is how life was every day, I could live to be 150."

You may have a place like that too. Maybe you're lucky enough to get there every year. Maybe you've only been there once in your life. But you remember it. And you remember what it felt like to be there.

The way we learn to manage the stress in our life is by giving ourselves moments that kindle that feeling. Of calm. Of quiet. Of peace.

If I could live in that delightful little California town where I take beach walks a handful of times a year, I would. But I can't. By some combination of choice and necessity, my life is elsewhere. Just like yours is.

What I had to learn over time was how to carve out a small space in my life where I could experience that tranquility for 15 or 20 minutes every day, rather than luxuriating in it for one week and then turning the wolves of stress loose on my defenseless brain as soon as I got home.

You can do the same, and you don't have to go anywhere special to achieve it. There are ways of taking your mind to a peaceful place without getting out of the chair you're sitting in right now.

THE CALMING POWER OF MUSIC

Let me suggest a couple of great ways to address your stress. One is listening to music. The other is meditation.

There's a reason these are two of the commonly recommended techniques for dealing with stress. They're readily available. They cost nothing. And for people with MCI, they work.

Consider the remarkable results from this study done at the University of West Virginia in 2018. It involved a group of 60 people with subjective cognitive decline who were asked to spend 12 minutes a day either listening to relaxing classical music or doing a form of meditation called Kirtan Kriya. After 12 weeks of doing this every day, they were told to continue the practice as often as they wanted to for another three months.

At the beginning of the study, their scores on memory tests fell in the range of mild cognitive impairment. When they were tested again after six months of meditating or listening to music, their scores had shot up. On average, they had returned to cognitively normal.

What's more, at the start of the study, 25 of the people were considered to be at high risk for dementia. By the end, all but seven of those people were no longer considered at high risk.

That's a result anyone with MCI would be glad to get. And it's something you can begin doing right now. Today. You can do your own experiment with 12 minutes a day of either music or meditation and see what it does for you.

I find that music, in particular, can be a good place for someone with MCI to start.

There are so many health behaviors that people find challenging to adopt, and they have all sorts of excuses for not trying. People tell me, "I can't exercise, it's too hard, it's too boring, I don't enjoy it. I can't eat this food. I can't eat that food. I hate the taste."

I have yet to have someone tell me, "I can't listen to music. I hate music."

There may be a particular type of music you don't like, the way I hate rap. But we all have some type of music we enjoy.

When I first wrote about this study, I got a lot of questions about exactly what classical music selections the people in the study listened to. But there wasn't a specific play list. They were given a choice among a variety of well-known composers like Mozart and Chopin. You may not like classical music anyway. You may prefer something else, and that's fine. Personally, I enjoy the classical composers, but I'm not a snob about it. I could listen to the Crosby, Stills & Nash version of "Blackbird" on a continuous loop for 12 minutes and be in cognitive heaven.

There's some musical choice that can do that for you. A neuropsychologist who has worked with MCI patients extensively for more than 20 years told me the music of Barbara Streisand often seems to work. "The Way We Were," anyone? How about Johnny Cash or Luther Vandross?

APPLYING THE BALM OF MEDITATION

Meditation is another option that any neurologist would highly recommend. Study after study has confirmed the cognitive benefits of meditation.

In the West Virginia study, the form of meditation offered was Kirtan Kriya. In brain health circles, it is one of the favorite forms of meditation, and there is an abundance of research to demonstrate its cognitive benefits.

The Alzheimer's Research & Prevention Foundation touts Kirtan Kriya as a nonreligious form of meditation that has been practiced for thousands of years. It involves chanting and finger movements and studies have shown practicing it for 12 minutes a day can reduce stress, "improve cognition and activate parts of the brain that are central to memory," the foundation says.

Another good choice for people with MCI is mindfulness meditation. You can practice mindfulness on your own, or through a program. The granddaddy of those programs is run by the Center for Mindfulness in Medicine, Health Care and Society at the UMass Medical Center, and you can learn more at its website.

If you are more interested in pursuing it on your own, a good way to get started is with this video, "How To Meditate In Twelve Minutes (Guided Meditation & Mindfulness Meditation for Beginners)" by Michael Sealey.

Another way to get started is by using the free version of the Headspace app. It will give you an introduction to the practice of mindfulness meditation, and then you can do it on your own, or continue with Headspace by paying a monthly subscription fee.

MORE WAYS TO TAMP DOWN STRESS

If you want to bring greater variety to the management of your stress, here's one more suggestion: spend more time outdoors.

There are lot of terms for it these days. Call it forest bathing. Or ecotherapy. Or a good old-fashioned walk in the woods. By any name, spending time outdoors reduces stress hormones in your body. Walking in the outdoors has proven so medicinal that some doctors are now writing prescriptions for it.

You don't have to escape to a national forest to get the benefit. A walk in a nearby park will do the trick. Just follow the advice of life coach Rasheed Ogunlaru, who says:

> *"Step outside for a while — calm your mind. It is better to hug a tree than to bang your head against a wall continually."*

78

Just remember, it's not about escaping stress. You can't. Stress is an inevitable part of life. It's about identifying the stresses in your life, and coping with them.

And there are so many ways to do that. Music. Meditation. Yoga. Breathing. Visualization. Muscle relaxation. Aromatherapy. Any of these techniques can help loosen the squeeze of stress upon your brain.

The very word stress is drawn from the Latin "stingere," which means to draw tight. Quell your stress. Calm your mind. Give your brain the moments of stillness it needs to help you fend off MCI.

TAKEAWAYS FROM CHAPTER 10

Prolonged, unaddressed stress can brutalize your brain. One neurologist calls it "a sledgehammer to the head."

The way we learn to manage the stress in our life is by giving ourselves moments that kindle a feeling of calm. Of quiet. Of peace.

Two of the best ways to address your stress are by listening to music or practicing meditation. They're readily available. They cost nothing. And for people with MCI, they work.

Other good ways to tamp down that stress include spending time outdoors, or using techniques such as breathing exercises, visualization, muscle relaxation or aromatherapy.

ONE ACTION, RIGHT NOW: Download the Headspace app and do a free, five-minute meditation every day for the next five days.

CHAPTER 11 — A Lighter Side To MCI

Nobody ever got a diagnosis of MCI and laughed. There's nothing funny about cognitive impairment.

Except, sometimes, there kind of is.

Every now and then, finding a little humor in MCI can help you in ways that even medicine can't.

When someone first gets that diagnosis of MCI, the common reactions are shock, dread, denial. But as you come to terms with this thing, there actually can be a lighter side to it.

I'm in a private Facebook group for people with MCI, and every day I see them sharing courage and compassion and kindness with each other. And humor. It's clearly part of what keeps them going.

"Humor definitely helps with the stress of living with MCI," says one woman. "It's always much better for me if I can laugh at something that I have done or said, rather than get upset about it."

She tells a story about the time she found a roll of masking tape in her freezer. "I looked at the masking tape and thought, 'Who could have done this?'" she recalls. "Then reality set in because I live alone, so no one could have done this except me. I just had to laugh."

Sven Svebak, a retired professor from the Norwegian University of Science and Technology, has spent more than 50 years studying the impact of humor on health and says it's a wonderful way to cope when you encounter bumps in the road of life.

"A sense of humor acts like shock absorbers in a car, a mental shock absorber in everyday life to help us cope better with a range of frustrations, hassles and irritations," he says.

Frustration. Hassle. Irritation. That barely begins to scratch the surface of what it's like to live with MCI. It's hard. But humor can help.

I'm not suggesting you should be happy to have MCI. I'm just encouraging you to find humor in it when you can.

Time and time again in the MCI group, I'll see somebody post something that made them laugh. And right away, other people will jump in and share their own humorous anecdotes. And at that point, the anecdote becomes the antidote.

There was the woman whose MCI makes it hard to find the right words. She was done listening to a CD and asked her husband to "push the erection button."

Or there was the man who couldn't seem to make a phone call to a friend. "I kept dialing the number and the call wouldn't go through," he says. "I finally realized what the problem was. I was trying to call him on the TV remote."

Sometimes, you just have to laugh.

"I can't imagine dealing with MCI — or life in general — without humor," one woman says. "Laughing with someone makes a connection. Most times I laugh with myself, outwardly or inwardly. It blows away the cobwebs and leaves a brightness. Maybe it's the pleasure hormones being released. Who cares? Humor is fun!"

ONE ACTION, RIGHT NOW: Pick one of the funniest movies you've ever seen, and watch it this evening.

CHAPTER 12 - Restorative Sleep

YOU SNOOZE, you lose.

What horrible advice that is — cognitively speaking. When it comes to brain health and memory, you lose when you *don't* snooze.

That's the reality we're finally waking up to.

We've known for a long time that exercise and diet are essential to cognition, and that if you don't keep your body moving and your brain properly fed, you're at risk for MCI and, eventually, dementia.

But sleep? Who needs sleep? From the time we're teenagers, we treat sleep as optional. When final exams come around, no problem. You pull an all-nighter. When it's crunch time on that big project at work, hey, something's got to give, so you burn the midnight oil.

There was a time when successful people skimped on sleep and wore it as a badge of honor. Dr. Rudolph Tanzi, a neurologist at the Harvard Medical School, was one of them. He used to brag about how well he could get by on three or four hours of sleep.

Except . . . he couldn't. None of us can. Sound, restorative sleep is one of the most fundamental needs of the human brain. Deprive yourself of that, and over a long enough period of time, the cognitive price can be enormous.

Dr. Tanzi, one of the nation's leading experts on Alzheimer's disease, understands that now. It's changed his entire attitude toward sleep.

"Religiously, I get 7 to 8 hours of sleep," he says, "because if you don't, you might as well be smoking cigarettes or sitting on the couch eating two bags of potato chips a night. It's the same thing."

That needs to be your attitude toward sleep, too.

If you're serious about defending your cognition, and giving yourself the best possible chance of slowing, halting or reversing MCI, you need a good night's sleep.

TWO COMMON MYTHS ABOUT SLEEP AND AGING

Somehow, we've convinced ourselves that as we get older, we don't need as much sleep as we used to. Or that sleeplessness is to be expected as we age, and that it's normal for older people to sleep fitfully and wake up on and off during the night.

Neither of those things is true. At any age, we need 7 to 8 hours of quality sleep to be physically and mentally at our best. And difficulty sleeping is not an inevitable consequence of getting old. Most often, it's a result of factors that can be addressed.

So let's help you sleep better, and let's make sure it's deep, restorative sleep. Because that's what your brain needs most.

You may have heard the term "sleep cycle." During the night, you have periods of lighter sleep and deeper sleep, and the deepest period of sleep is referred to as REM or "rapid eye movement" sleep. You may go through four to six sleep cycles over the course of the night, and REM sleep — which may last anywhere from 10 minutes to an hour during each cycle — is the one that matters most to cognition.

New research tells us that three important things are going on in your brain during deep sleep:

· It's the time when a clear, clean solution circulates through the brain, washing away toxins. Think of it like taking your brain through the car wash.

- It's also the only time when the brain does not produce beta-amyloid, the so-called "plaque" that accumulates in the brain of people with Alzheimer's disease.
- Deep sleep is when new memories are moved to regions of the brain where they are stored. Without this activity, your ability to preserve memories is compromised.

THE PERNICIOUS THREAT OF SLEEP APNEA

If you're having trouble sleeping, there are many possible reasons why. One of the most pernicious is a sleep disorder called sleep apnea. It's a common problem, particularly among older men or people who are overweight, and it's strongly associated with MCI.

Sleep apnea occurs when soft tissue at the back of the mouth and throat blocks the airway. People with sleep apnea often snore loudly and may wake up hundreds of times a night without realizing it. That robs their brain of REM sleep and invites serious cognitive problems.

I shared this statistic earlier, but it's so jarring that I want to remind you of it again.

Researchers scoured the medical histories of some 2,500 people between the ages of 55 and 90 to see what role sleep played in their risk of cognitive impairment.

- For those who had sleep apnea or some other sleep disorder, the average age they developed MCI was 77.
- For those with no sleep disorder, the onset of MCI didn't come until

an average age of 90.

And then there's Per Laursen, who was an unlikely candidate for cognitive problems at any age. He didn't get MCI at the age of 90. Or at the age of 77. He was diagnosed at the ripe young age of 53, and his tale is a cautionary one.

Per Laursen hails from Denmark (but he's not the world-class Danish darts player of the same name). Professionally, Per taught coping and stress management skills at a major global corporation. He was physically active, ate well and kept his mind cognitively stimulated. He speaks two languages, and he's not only a musician, he makes his own guitars.

In short, he was a model of brain health in every way but one, yet that vulnerability was enough to tip the balance against him.

I met Per after doing a video on the different ways that people halt or reverse their MCI, and how to "round up the usual suspects" — lack of exercise, lousy diet, unaddressed stress and poor sleep. He contacted me the same day and said, "I'm one of your usual suspects."

Per, now 70, was diagnosed with MCI by a neurologist in 2003. At that time, MCI was presumed to automatically lead to Alzheimer's, and there wasn't much to be done about it. Per wasn't willing to accept that. He chose to defend his cognition.

"My wife brought me finally to my GP and she suggested a sleep study in the hospital," Per recalls. "I got a nightly sleep test, and the first thing that the doctor said in the morning was, 'Why didn't you come five years before, Per?' The (problem) for me was Obstructive Sleep Apnea and the lack of oxygen in the brain, leading to MCI. If I had come before, I could have avoided MCI. But I didn't."

Fortunately, even back then, sleep apnea could be addressed. Per got the proper treatment and devoted himself to brain health in other ways, eventually writing a book about it.

I asked him if he's been able to halt or reverse his MCI. "I have, I certainly have," he told me. "Over the years, I seemed to work it out, and got gradually better functioning, day by day and year by year. Now I can read and write again, at a level close to pre-MCI."

For far too long, sleep apnea was the silent stalker of an aging brain, but the word is out now. Screening for it has become common, and if you haven't been screened, you should be.

If you suspect you might have sleep apnea, don't ignore it. You'll find everything you need to know about identifying and treating it here.

TIPS TO GET A GOOD NIGHT'S REST

Sleep disorders are far from the only impediment to a good night's rest. There are so many other possible causes — and so many people who fall victim to them.

A study done several years ago found 42 percent of people over the age of 65 reported some difficulty in falling asleep or staying asleep. The percentage is probably higher now because of the time spent staring at the screens of electronic devices, which can disrupt our rest.

Among the more common causes are alcohol, depression, caffeine or pain caused by a medical condition such as arthritis. All can be addressed and if they are, you can get better sleep.

There also is a lot of good information available these days on how to improve your "sleep hygiene." These are simple, practical ways to improve your bedtime routine and sleep more soundly as a result. That can include

• avoiding eating or exercise in the last two to three hours before you go to bed.

• not drinking coffee or other beverages with caffeine after midafternoon.

· not smoking. If you're a smoker, your body experiences nicotine withdrawal during the night, which interrupts your sleep.

· darkening your bedroom by closing the blinds, and setting the room temperature so it's neither hot nor cold.

· trying to get to bed and get up at the same time every day.

· considering replacing your pillows and/or mattress if they've become uncomfortable to sleep on.

· not watching TV in bed, and not having electronics (such as your phone) in the bedroom. Electronic devices emit a blue light that interferes with your ability to sleep.

· not lying awake if you can't fall asleep. Get out of bed, and then go back to bed later.

· avoiding napping during the day if you're not sleeping well at night.

You can learn more about sleep and sleep disorders by visiting the website of the American Sleep Association.

The National Sleep Foundation also is an excellent resource, and you can learn more by checking out its website.

Are you determined to defend your cognition? Then let sleep be your ally.

You want night to be the time when you close your eyes and let deep, restorative sleep do the work for you.

As Akiroq Brost says: "As important as it is to have a plan for doing work, it is perhaps more important to have a plan for rest, relaxation, self-care, and sleep."

TAKEAWAYS FROM CHAPTER 12

Sound, restorative sleep is one of the most fundamental needs of the

human brain. Deprive yourself of adequate sleep, and cognition can suffer.

We need seven to eight hours of quality sleep a night at any age. Difficulty sleeping is not an inevitable result of getting older. Most often, it's a result of factors that can be addressed.

Sleep apnea is a common sleep disorder that can result in serious cognitive impairment. It particularly is seen in older men or people who are overweight, and it's strongly associated with MCI.

There are simple, practical ways to improve your bedtime routine and sleep more soundly.

ONE ACTION, RIGHT NOW: Beginning today, don't have your phone in the bedroom with you when you go to sleep at night.

CHAPTER 13 – Train Your Brain

HOW AM I doing?

People with MCI ask that question a lot. They want to know what's going on with their cognition. Are they getting better? Are they getting worse? They wonder, they worry, they obsess endlessly about it.

Yet they're often left guessing. They can go months, even years, without knowing whether their cognition has changed in any measurable way.

But that doesn't have to be you. If you really want to know, you can find out. With online cognitive testing that's available these days, you can measure your cognition as often as you want and track your score over time, so you know how you're progressing.

For people with mild cognitive impairment, that's a game-changer.

Not just because it can satisfy your curiosity or calm your worries. But because it makes you a more effective manager of your own health behavior, letting you measure your progress to better understand what is or isn't working for you.

SELF-TESTING OFFERS AN ANSWER

Testing your cognition at home isn't something you do instead of being tested by a doctor. You need to be seen by a doctor, and tested and diagnosed by a doctor, so you know what you're dealing with and what your treatment should be.

When a doctor tests you, they use a tool like the MoCA. (There are other tests, such as the MMSE or the Mini-Cog, but I mention the MoCA because it's particularly sensitive to detecting MCI.) The doctor gives you the test, scores it and then interprets the results for you. Ideally, you're also referred to a neuropsychologist for much more extensive testing.

But at some point, the doctors are done with you.

So you go home. And now it's just you and your MCI. What then?

Well, you get to work. You begin to defend your cognition, by doing the things your doctors recommend and the things we know will give you the best chance of slowing, halting or reversing cognitive decline. You get your body moving. You eat better. You give meditation or yoga a try. You pay attention to how much sleep you're getting.

And you spend an awful lot of time asking yourself, is any of this stuff doing me any good? Am I getting better? Or at least not getting worse?

That's when you might turn to self-testing and brain training for an answer.

YES, THERE'S A TEST FOR THAT

Of all the innovations in health care, the ability of patients to perform simple medical tests on themselves at home is one of the most revolutionary. It makes them better managers of their own care, and it leads to better outcomes.

If you have hypertension, your doctor can give you a blood pressure monitor to use at home. When you're checking your blood pressure on a daily basis, you can do a better job of controlling it.

All sorts of home testing kits are available these days. Want to know if you're pregnant? There's a test for that. Want to measure your cholesterol level or your body fat or the electrical activity in your heart? You can test any of those things at home.

But what if you want to know whether your cognition is getting better or worse?

Try brain training. It doesn't just give you an answer. It actually gives you a better chance of getting the answer you want.

In fact, brain training is one of the best weapons we have against MCI, which makes me wonder why more people with cognitive impairment don't take advantage of it.

HARNESSING THE POWER OF NEUROGENESIS

Let me clarify what I mean by brain training.

There are all sorts of "brain games" — from Sudoku to crossword puzzles to Words with Friends — and they're OK. There's no reason not to play those games, if you enjoy them.

But "brain training" refers to something else. It's a form of exercise for your brain that's developed by neurologists specifically for the purpose of improving cognitive function and reducing the risk of Alzheimer's.

Brain training is available online through such programs as BrainHQ, Lumosity, Dakim or Cogstate. These are names you may already know, particularly BrainHQ or Lumosity. Your doctor may even have recommended one of them to you.

You do these cognitive exercises on your computer or phone. You play them like you would a game, but they offer a benefit that so-called brain games don't. And here's why: They trigger what's called "neurogenesis." That's a fancy scientific term for what happens when you grow new brain cells or new neural connections, and it's a concept anyone with MCI ought to know and take advantage of. Here are answers to some questions you might have about that.

If neurogenesis is so good for my brain, how do I get it?

Neurogenesis occurs when you force your brain to figure out how to do something that's new and a little bit difficult. That stimulates your brain to generate more neurons and neural pathways.

But how does that help my brain?

It makes the brain stronger and more resilient, and it allows other parts of your brain to do a better job of stepping in and compensating for whatever is going wrong in the part of your brain that's being affected by MCI. We've talked a lot in this book about tipping the cognitive balance. This is one way to tip that balance back in your brain's favor.

Can't I do that by playing Sudoku or doing crossword puzzles?

Unfortunately, no. As you play those games over and over, your brain becomes too familiar with them. The more you play them, the more proficient you become, but you're just getting better at that particular game. It doesn't translate into a broader cognitive benefit.

So what should I try instead?

Anything novel and challenging can trigger neurogenesis. If you're right-handed, try something with your left hand. Or take a different route to drive home. Or teach yourself to juggle. Or take up a new hobby, or learn how to fix a leaking faucet, or play fantasy football, or grow orchids.

But what science has shown us is that for people with mild cognitive impairment, doing brain training can be one of the best answers.

Brain training can boost cognition. It can reduce the risk of dementia. And here's one more big plus: It can serve as a form of cognitive testing, allowing you to track how your brain is doing over time.

THE RIGHT WAY TO TRAIN YOUR BRAIN

In the pantheon of cognitive protectors, brain training doesn't always get its due, but it belongs right up there with exercise, diet, stress management and restorative sleep.

It's been studied extensively over the past decade, and based purely on research results, it's one of the single best ways for people with MCI to improve cognitive function and reduce the risk of dementia. That's according to the National Academies of Sciences, Engineering and Medicine, which issued a white paper on the subject in 2017.

The National Academies said the three best opportunities to slow cognitive impairment and prevent the onset of dementia can be found in

- physical activity/exercise,
- blood pressure management for people with hypertension, and
- cognitive training

And although it spoke generally about brain training, it particularly referenced a brain exercise that's available in the BrainHQ program.

Among brain-training programs, BrainHQ has emerged as the clear leader. There's some evidence to support other brain-training programs as well. But I recommend BrainHQ because the evidence behind it is so overwhelming, and because of the number of BrainHQ studies involving people with MCI and the consistent benefit it has shown for people with that degree of cognitive impairment.

If you decide to try BrainHQ, you can sign up for it online and start with a free trial. Once the trial is over, you pay a monthly fee to continue, which is true of other brain-training programs as well. (Please note: BrainHQ has proven to be so effective that many insurers now cover the cost of it for people with cognitive impairment.)

Once you're signed up, you can choose the exercises you do, or you can use the "personal trainer," which will assess your cognitive strengths and weaknesses and design a training program for you.

For someone with mild cognitive impairment, two good exercises to begin with are the ones called Double Decision and Hawkeye.

A major long-term study showed Double Decision can reduce the risk for dementia by 48 percent up to 10 years after the training. Across all the possible treatments for MCI, you'll be hard pressed to find something that offers a potential benefit as good as that.

Based on recent research done specifically on people with MCI, you may also want to try the BrainHQ exercises called Eye for Detail, Target Tracker and Visual Sweeps.

BrainHQ suggests that you train 10 or 20 a minutes a day five times a week, or you can shoot for a 30-minute training session three times a week.

These games can feel like a form of tough love for your brain. I've had people with MCI tell me that the BrainHQ exercises are "too hard." In reality, they are designed to be hard, but just the right amount of hard to trigger neurogenesis for you.

It reminds me of a friend who once jokingly said to me, "Yeah, I tried lifting weights, but I didn't like it. They were too heavy."

That's what you have to understand about BrainHQ. It's not a game or a lighthearted leisure activity. It's a form of cognitive strength training.

The program assesses your capabilities and continually adjust the degree of difficulty to keep you challenged. Don't let it frustrate you, and don't feel like a failure. View it as a good, vigorous workout for your mind that can help your brain start working better again over time.

TRACK HOW YOUR COGNITION IS TRENDING

There's one other thing brain training offers you over time. It's a legitimate form of cognitive testing that allows you to see how much benefit you're getting and what direction your cognition is trending in.

Whether you use BrainHQ or a program like Dakim or Lumosity or Cogstate, you earn points or stars for the exercises you do. But they also rank you against other people your age who play the same games, and give you a percentile score.

So if, for instance, BrainHQ puts you in the 50th percentile, that means you rank in the top half for people your age.

That percentile ranking is what you want to track. Not on a daily basis, but over a longer period of time — maybe every three months, or every six months.

This is a tip that Dr. Dale Bredesen teaches us in his book, *The End of Alzheimer's,* and it's an important one.

Dr. Bredesen says this percentile ranking is a valid form of cognitive testing, just like the MMSE or MoCA, those tests that doctors use. He tells his patients the "target value" is ranking above the 50th percentile for your age, and improving as you continue to practice.

As soon as you begin brain training, you want to note what your percentile is for your age group. It may tell you that you're at the 45th percentile. Or the 53rd percentile, or the 61st percentile. Whatever that number is, it becomes your baseline score.

From there, you want to watch how your percentile score changes over time. That way, you never have to ask, is my cognition getting better? Is it getting worse? The trajectory of your percentile will tell you.

For someone who is committed to defending their cognition, that can be invaluable. It can show you how well what you are doing is working, or tell you when it's time to try other things.

If the percentile score shows your cognition is edging in the wrong direction, you're better off knowing that, so you can reassess and try other approaches.

If your percentile score is on the rise, then you can double down on whatever you're doing, knowing you're on the right track.

A BRAIN-TRAINING SUCCESS STORY

Steve Raymond, a 67-year-old retired nursing home administrator from Maine, is one of my favorite examples of someone who used BrainHQ to help pull himself out of cognitive decline — and track his success along the way.

Raymond was still working at the time, running a senior retirement community on the coast of Maine, when his memory began to fail him in a way he found alarming.

"There were a couple of times when I became lost in familiar places, and that one really freaked me out because I understood the significance of that," he says. "It was other things, too. I've always been a voracious reader, but I found I was avoiding reading, because after a few pages, I'd lose the thread of it and get so frustrated."

Raymond knew what he needed to do to defend his cognition, and he had some strengths in those areas already.

"Exercise is something I've always done easily; I love exercise," he says. "I eat well, most of the time. I've been working with nutritional ketosis for quite a while. Social engagement is not an issue for me. I'm a natural engager."

Still, his cognition was floundering, so Raymond committed to what he calls "optimum brain health." That included a vigorous brain-training program, using BrainHQ.

Early on, he recalls scoring in the 61st percentile for his age. That's above the 50th percentile that Dr. Bredesen recommends as a target, but Raymond knew his cognitive abilities wouldn't have to slip much further to fall into the 50s, or lower. He continued to train his brain in earnest.

As I was finishing this book, I checked back in with Raymond. He flipped open his laptop and proudly showed me his dashboard in BrainHQ. Even though he'd recently taken a break from training, his score sat at an impressive 86th percentile for his age. His score for navigation skills — 90th percentile. His score for people skills — 92nd percentile.

But here's what matters most: Those gains translated into noticeably better cognitive performance in his daily life. He reports no problems with getting lost in familiar places. "That hasn't happened to me at all recently," he says. His reading comprehension is back where it used to be, too.

Raymond serves on community boards, and says at his lowest point, "I would lose track of the conversation and not be able to keep up with what's going on." Not anymore. "Now, I have the feeling that, wow, I'm tracking this so much better," he says.

Brain training was just one part of the answer for Raymond. But he says it accelerated his cognitive recovery like nothing else seemed to.

"With BrainHQ, I was consciously aware of the improvement; I felt it quite definitely," Raymond says.

"I wouldn't put it all on BrainHQ, but I want to give credit where credit is due," he says. "Yes, I was doing other things, but I feel BrainHQ made a pretty definitive difference on top of what else I was doing."

TAKEAWAYS FROM CHAPTER 13

With online cognitive testing that's available these days, you can measure your cognition and track your score over time, so you know how you're progressing.

The ability of patients to perform simple medical tests on themselves at home is revolutionary. It makes them better managers of their own care, and it leads to better outcomes.

Brain training is a form of exercise for your brain that's developed by neurologists specifically to improve cognitive function and reduce the risk of dementia.

Brain training has been scientifically shown to benefit cognition, and by tracking your percentile score over time, you get an accurate measure of how your cognition is trending.

ONE ACTION, RIGHT NOW: Sign up for the free version of BrainHQ, play the game called "Double Decision" for a week and see what your percentile is for your age group.

CHAPTER 14 — Mercury And Mold

WHEN YOU were a kid and had a cavity, you went to the dentist for a filling.

Do you know what that filling consisted of? Silver, partly. But also tin, and about 50 percent mercury.

Here's what Dr. Mary Kay Ross wants to know: "Who had the great idea of putting a toxic metal — mercury — in our mouths as children?" she asks.

That may have nothing to do with the cognitive problems you're experiencing now. But it's a reminder of how oblivious we are to the environmental hazards we come in contact with every day and the potential harm they can do to our brain.

Mold. Fungi. Toxins. Heavy metals.

They're everywhere. We are exposed to them throughout our lives, and Dr. Ross says they can exact a cognitive toll.

"From a toxic perspective, we all have the responsibility of knowing the dangers we put our body in," she says. "We have created a world that is incredibly toxic. We don't realize all the things that add to our toxic burden. But eventually you reach a tipping point and become ill."

Dr. Ross, founder and CEO of the Brain Health & Research Institute in Seattle, is one of the nation's leading authorities on the role that mold, toxins and heavy metals can play in MCI and dementia.

I asked her where mold or heavy metals fit in the overall risk for cognitive impairment.

"Here's what I tell patients," Dr. Ross says. "Chronic illnesses do not just happen. They occur over a period of time and there's always an underlying reason, related to genetics, lifestyle and an acute exposure that is the tipping point."

"STOP EATING THAT FISH!"

When Dr. Ross told me that, I immediately thought of Miriam, because it describes her experience exactly.

I shared Miriam's story with you earlier in the book. She threw herself into diet and exercise, and those changes did her a lot of good. Getting therapy and learning how to manage her stress made a difference, too. She was doing better, but she still wasn't where she wanted to be cognitively. Something was missing.

For Miriam, the final turning point came when she was referred to an enthusiastic young neurologist, just out of medical school and full of fresh ideas.

"After I started seeing her, she began running all these different tests," Miriam says. "She told me, 'I have some blood work I want to do on you.' It's called a dementia profile. She did my blood work in April (2019). Because I was eating fish all the time, she wanted to be sure my mercury levels and my lead levels were OK."

The test results came back and showed there indeed was a problem. Miriam had high levels of mercury, not to mention arsenic. Her neurologist moved immediately to address the problem. "She told me, 'Stop eating that fish,'" Miriam says.

Her neurologist predicted it would take six months to a year for Miriam to flush the mercury out of her system. But a month later, she says, "my brain was clear."

Finally, after more than four years of effort, Miriam had finally tipped the cognitive balance back in her brain's favor. The next time she saw her neurologist, she tested cognitively normal.

That's the happy ending anyone with MCI would want, but there was a moral to Miriam's story, and it wasn't lost on me. The day she told me about her mercury poisoning, I stopped eating tuna.

HOW MERCURY GETS STORED IN YOUR BRAIN

When you're trying to eat in a more brain-healthy way, one of the first things you're told is to eat less red meat and more fish. And especially cold-water fish such as tuna or salmon, which are high in the omega-3 fatty acids that are so nourishing to cognition.

That's what Miriam did. That's what I did, too. I had been eating tuna once or twice a week. Tuna sandwiches. Tuna salad. Sushi.

What neither Miriam nor I took into account was the risk of mercury that comes with consumption of tuna. According to the World Health Organization, exposure to mercury can cause serious health problems, and the primary way we end up with mercury in our brain is from eating fish or shellfish that are tainted with it. The greatest risk comes from larger, predatory fish such as tuna or swordfish.

Miriam found this out the hard way, and I benefitted from her experience. I figured, why take the risk? Better not to eat tuna at all.

Occasionally, though, I wondered if I was overreacting. So when I met Dr. Ross, that was one of the first questions I asked her. Was it the right choice to give up eating tuna?

"I would tell you that's very smart," she said. "I don't eat any of those large fish for the same reasons. I think mercury toxicity is a big problem.

We store them in fat. They get stored in our brain."

She does recommend fish as a brain-healthy choice but encourages her patients to stick with smaller cold-water fish that are sometimes referred to as the "SMASH" fish: sardines, mackerel, anchovies, wild-caught salmon and herring.

HOUSES BUILT OUT OF "MOLD FOOD"

Dr. Ross also has deep concern about the potential cognitive impact of household mold, and that's based not just on her professional training and research, but also on personal experience.

She calls mold toxicity one of the biggest drivers of cognitive loss. "It releases mycotoxins, nanoparticles that we can inhale and they can become lodged in our lungs and even enter our brains," she says. "They are small enough to pass through the blood-brain barrier and lodge in our brain. People can develop cancers, they can develop lung disease, they can develop Alzheimer's."

Dr. Ross describes mold as "nature's great disintegrator," and in the wild, it does its work without posing any particular threat to human health.

"But mold becomes a really big problem when it's inside your home," she says. "Unfortunately, we build our houses out of mold food. Mold loves drywall."

Dr. Ross tells the story of one family where the mother has dementia, and now the daughter is experiencing declining health, including memory loss. And the common denominator appears to be mold toxicity.

"My patient is the daughter, who has mild cognitive impairment and many other health problems, and it's related to the mold in the mother's house," Dr. Ross says. "At the end of the day, that's probably why the mother is dying of Alzheimer's. It's really scary."

More than a decade ago, Dr Ross had her own health scare due to mold, and it changed the course of her career.

She was an emergency room doctor working at a trauma center in Savannah, Georgia, when she was beset by a baffling array of illnesses that included arthritis, a heart condition and respiratory problems. "It became so bad, I almost had to go on disability," she says.

Dr. Ross sought out specialists, including a leading infectious disease doctor in New York, but no one could explain her failing health. She began looking for her own answers.

"I couldn't sleep for two years, so I would sit up and do research," she says. "I eventually realized a lot of these symptoms I was having led back to mold."

What she eventually discovered was that the drain in her shower had developed a leak, and the dripping water led to an ugly infestation of mold hidden behind a wall in her home. "You couldn't see it, but oh my gosh, the wall was black," she says.

Dr. Ross moved out of her house the same day the mold was discovered, and almost immediately her health began to improve. But even as she recovered, the experience called her in a new direction professionally.

She spent two years retraining in functional medicine, and in 2012, she launched The Institute for Personalized Medicine, where she became a leader in research on molds, toxins, fungi, and heavy metals, focusing on how they contribute to neurodegenerative diseases.

BE INTENTIONAL ABOUT AVOIDING TOXINS

In the case of Dr. Ross, the exposure to mold hidden behind the walls in her home was the trigger, but genetics played a role, too. She says approximately 25 percent of people have a genetic susceptibility to biotoxins, including mold, and that leaves them vulnerable to chronic illness — including cognitive impairment or Alzheimer's — if they have exposure to mold at home or their workplace.

For these people, she says, lifestyle changes such as diet, exercise and stress reduction can be helpful and are recommended. But healthy habits by themselves won't be enough.

"If you live in a moldy environment and start to develop cognitive issues, none of those are going to be a perfect cure if your home is toxic," she says. "I will support you with the pillars (of brain health), and you can have a chef and a nutritionist and a health coach, and you will get somewhat better. But the day we discover the true tipping point of your disease, that is the determining factor. That is what really makes the difference."

That was true for Miriam. It may or may not be true for you.

To defend your cognition is to understand the possible threats and guard yourself against them. The traditional treatment of mild cognitive impairment and dementia typically did not consider mold or mercury as a possible cause or contributor, and Dr. Dale Bredesen insists that we can no longer afford to overlook the role that "chronic, mild toxicity" can potentially play in cognitive decline.

"We've had to drag people kicking and screaming into the 21st Century to recognize that this has been an issue," he says. "You have to look at this. If you find the toxin, when you address it, people get better. This is a critical thing to look at."

Dr. Bredesen recommends anyone over the age of 45 who is experiencing cognitive problems, including memory loss, should consider being tested for exposure to mercury or mycotoxins.

It's something to be aware of and talk to your doctor about.

If you get tested, and the results are negative, at least that's one risk you can cross off your list. It's certainly better to know your status than to have mercury or mycotoxins floating around in your brain and not be aware of it.

It's also important to be more intentional about avoiding foods or products that contain mercury, lead, arsenic or other toxins. According to Dr. Ross, that can include everything from lipstick and weed killer to apple juice, rice and, yes, even tuna.

Sorry, Charlie.

TAKEAWAYS FROM CHAPTER 14

Mold. Fungi. Toxins. Heavy metals. We are exposed to them throughout life, and they can exact a cognitive toll.

Exposure to mercury can cause serious health problems, and the primary way we end up with mercury in our brain is from eating fish or shellfish that are tainted with it.

Household mold can cause cognitive loss. Approximately 25 percent of people have a genetic susceptibility to biotoxins, including mold, and that leaves them vulnerable to cognitive impairment.

Dr. Dale Bredesen recommends anyone over the age of 45 who is experiencing cognitive problems should consider being tested for exposure to mercury or mycotoxins.

ONE ACTION, RIGHT NOW: Read this article from the National Institutes of Health on ways to minimize exposure to toxins. gocogno.com/go/toxins

CHAPTER 15 — Joining A Clinical Trial

IF YOU could go to an elite medical clinic, be seen by top doctors, have access to cutting-edge treatment, and it cost you little or nothing, does that sound like a good deal to you?

That opportunity exists, by enrolling in a clinical trial. It's something anyone with mild cognitive impairment ought to at least consider.

These are exciting times in the search for more effective treatments for mild cognitive impairment and dementia. Our ability to say with confidence that it is possible to halt or reverse MCI is due to the breakthroughs we've seen in one study after another over the past two or three years.

So think for a moment about those who volunteered for that research. They were people with MCI, just like you. Without them, these advances would not have occurred. You owe them a debt of thanks.

And you owe it to yourself to consider joining their ranks, if the opportunity is available and it's the right choice for you. As one patient put it:

"I intend to try by all means available to get better, or at least not to get any worse than I am right now, so I feel that I have nothing to lose by joining a study."

These days, the field of research is rich with choices. There are major studies looking at how to combine lifestyle improvements in ways that provide the greatest benefit for people with MCI. There are highly anticipated studies for promising new drugs that specifically target MCI.

And, of course, there is a multibillion-dollar research effort to find desperately needed treatments for Alzheimer's disease and other forms of dementia. As disappointing as past defeats have been, scientists have learned much from them. The studies of today are better designed, and the drugs and other approaches are more promising.

Any one of these current studies could be the blockbuster treatment we've been waiting for. And you could potentially help make that happen, benefitting both yourself and future generations in the process.

Plus, there are a whole set of secondary benefits that come from being evaluated for a clinical trial, even if you never actually join one. That's why it's at least worth looking into. And believe me, they're looking for you.

THEY'RE LOOKING FOR SOMEONE LIKE YOU

The whole emphasis of dementia research has shifted toward mild cognitive impairment in recent years. Perhaps one reason past experiments have failed is because the drug was given too late. By then, too much damage already had been done to the brain. That's the theory, anyway. The idea is to get the drug to the person sooner, either at the MCI stage or even before that.

So people with mild cognitive impairment have become prime candidates for the latest studies. Perhaps your doctor has talked to you about enrolling in a clinical trial. But if not, you can ask your doctor about that, or seek out your own opportunity.

If you decide to be evaluated for a clinical trial, you have everything to gain.

Simply going to a clinic and getting screened for a study is your gateway to a level of advanced medical care for cognitive impairment. The people who run these clinics are tops in their field, so they're up on all the latest treatments and techniques.

Among other things, being screened for a study can act as a de facto second opinion. Researchers at these clinics will look carefully at you. Their job is to find exactly the right patients for whatever clinical trial they're looking to fill. So they have a vested interest in understanding your condition and making sure you weren't misdiagnosed or that the doctors didn't miss something that can be addressed through traditional medicine that's already available.

If you don't qualify for any trial they're doing right now, you're still way ahead of the game for reasons that include the following:

- They now have a baseline measure of your cognition, so if you go back and get tested every year, they can detect any changes in your memory.
- If a clinical trial comes along in the future that might be ideal for you, they'll let you know.
- If they spot anything your doctors haven't, they can refer you to a good doctor in your area to get it addressed. Or it may be something they can treat you for right there at their clinic, even without you joining a study.

If you are a potential match for a current trial, you'll get a much more thorough workup, including sophisticated tests that otherwise might not be available to you. And this will cost you little or nothing. Most of it is provided free of charge.

WHAT A CLINICAL TRIAL OFFERS

It's not easy to get into a clinical trial, and if you enroll in one, it's a real commitment. You need a study partner, usually a family member, to join you in the process.

You have to be faithful in taking the medication or other treatment on the schedule they set for you over the entire course of the study period, which can be months.

You will need to travel to the clinic on an occasional basis for checkups. You will undergo testing periodically. There may be risks that you need to fully understand and be willing to accept.

So being part of a study will ask a lot of you. But it also will offer a lot to you.

You will be advancing a treatment that has already shown real potential and might be "the one" — that next breakthrough that we know is coming at some point. If it works, others still might have to wait years to receive it while it undergoes regulatory approval, but you're getting it now. That's the most optimistic outcome, but any treatment far enough along to qualify for a Phase II or Phase III study has that potential.

If the medication shows benefit, you can receive it even if you start out in the placebo group. The way clinical trials work, some people get the medicine and some get a placebo. That is assigned randomly, and during the trial, you don't know if you're getting the real drug or not. People sometimes are reluctant to join a trial because they feel if they get the placebo, they're wasting their time. Please don't let that stop you from participating. If a drug shows a result and you were taking the placebo, the researchers can ask for approval to start giving you the drug after you're done taking the placebo.

You're playing a part in finding a cure sooner. The biggest challenge we face right now in curing dementia is a chronic shortage of volunteers to take part in studies. A clinical trial can take years to complete, and the biggest reason for that is how long it takes to enroll enough people in the study. Experts say getting these studies fully enrolled at a faster pace could cut years off the time it takes to find treatments for Alzheimer's.

You get the satisfaction of knowing you're doing something important that can benefit your children and grandchildren. Anyone who enters a clinical trial hopes to be part of history, and get what turns out to be that blockbuster drug. But they understand that may or may not happen. They're hopeful, but it's not their primary motivation. What really drives most people is a sense of altruism. They know we need a cure, and they know they're making a valuable contribution that will benefit others. Future generations will owe a huge debt of gratitude to those who are helping to advance the science now, and you could be one of those people.

"DO I HAVE ALZHEIMER'S OR DON'T I?"

There is one other opportunity that a clinical trial may represent for you, and it's a huge one.

It's the chance to potentially answer the burning question that anyone with mild cognitive impairment has. Do I have Alzheimer's or don't I?

You may have a family history of Alzheimer's, and if so, you can't help but be worried. Your doctor may have told you that the underlying cause of your MCI is suspected Alzheimer's. Or maybe your doctor has suggested it isn't.

But most people who have MCI live without knowing for sure. Even though the answer is available, they don't have access to it.

In very recent years, tests have emerged that can tell pretty definitively whether a person has Alzheimer's by measuring the amount of beta-amyloid plaques in their brain. But these tests can be invasive and expensive and usually aren't covered by insurance, so most people with MCI don't get them.

So the specter of Alzheimer's hangs over them, and some deal with that better than others. Some people want to know, especially now that it's possible to find out. If you are one of those people, that can be another compelling reason to consider a clinical trial.

These days, enrolling in a study has become one of the best ways to get what's called an amyloid PET scan. This scan, which costs thousands of dollars, is the surest way we have to accurately diagnose Alzheimer's in someone with MCI. Depending on the clinical trial you're being considered for, you may be able to get a PET scan at no cost to you as part of the evaluation for the study.

Is it Alzheimer's? If you're determined to know, then volunteering for a study can potentially be a way to get the answer.

FINDING A CLINICAL TRIAL NEAR YOU

If you decide to look into a clinical trial, there are three good ways to go about it.

The first is to talk to your primary care doctor or neurologist. They may be able to recommend one to you, or watch for a new one that comes along and might be a good fit for you.

The next place I'd encourage you to turn to would be the Global Alzheimer's Platform, a coalition of more than 80 of the leading medical clinics in the United States and Canada. This first-of-its kind network, launched in 2016, has brought a more agile, entrepreneurial, fast-moving approach to the search for a cure.

Its goal is simple. It seeks to speed up the discovery of innovative therapies for Alzheimer's by reducing the time and cost of clinical trials.

This alliance includes such major universities as Stanford, Georgetown, Northwestern and Emory, as well as the Mayo Clinic and the Cleveland Clinic.

These cutting-edge centers of research are seeking what they call "citizen scientists" to help them find a cure sooner. They are particularly looking for people with MCI to volunteer for clinical trials, and they welcome you to contact them. You can use the GAP-Net locator search tool to see if there's a center near you and learn how to contact it.

If you live near one of these research sites, that represents an opportunity to enter a world of high-quality care, much of which will be offered to you for free.

They can evaluate you, match you with a clinical trial if you qualify for one, and educate you on all the other things you can do to defend your cognition, through their Acti-V8 Your Brain Program, which emphasizes the eight pillars of brain health that anyone with MCI needs to know and incorporate in their life.

If there isn't a GAPNet site near you, there still may be other clinical trials available in your area. To find them, you can go to the website of the National Institute on Aging, where they offer a search tool for clinical trials devoted to mild cognitive impairment and dementia. It's available here.

Always keep in mind, joining a clinical trial is additive. It's not something you do instead of addressing healthy habits like exercise, diet, sleep and stress reduction. It's something you want to do in concert with those efforts, to give yourself the best possible chance of slowing, halting or reversing your cognitive impairment.

You're under no obligation to volunteer for a clinical trial, and don't feel like you're failing yourself if you don't find a way to enroll in one. You may not match the criteria. You may live too far from a study location. You may look into it and decide it's just not something you want to do.

But you owe it to yourself to consider it. Whether you simply get that initial evaluation or take it all the way through to enrollment in a clinical trial, you will find there are so many upsides for you all along the way.

Even if you don't end up taking part in a study, the process of merely being evaluated for one can bring you closer to your goal of slowing, halting or reversing your MCI.

Karen Watson, a woman from Daytona Beach, Florida, who joined a clinical trial at a GAPNet site, sums it up perfectly.

"I would say look at the bigger picture," she says. "The benefits of participating go far beyond any medication you receive. We're doing this for future generations. Besides, if you can do something to stop your own memory loss, why wouldn't you do it?"

TAKEAWAYS FROM CHAPTER 15

You owe it to yourself to consider joining a clinical trial, if the opportunity is available and it's the right choice for you.

The whole emphasis of dementia research has shifted toward mild cognitive impairment. The idea is to get the drug to the person sooner, either at the MCI stage or even before that.

Simply going to a clinic and getting screened for a study is your gateway to a level of advanced medical care for cognitive impairment.

By enrolling in a clinical trial, you will be advancing a treatment that

has already shown real potential and might be "the one."

Enrolling in a study can be one potential way to get an amyloid PET scan, which can detect whether you do or don't have Alzheimer's.

ONE ACTION, RIGHT NOW: Use the site locator tool to see if there is a GAP-Net research center near you.

CHAPTER 16 — The Go Cogno Credo

I WISH that I — or a doctor, or some scientist or savant — could tell you right now exactly what to do in order to defend your cognition. But the "what" is different for every single person, based on their unique strengths and vulnerabilities, and that is a process of discovery.

Still, I have seen people with MCI succeed, and I've seen how they've done it, and I can tell you this much. There are ways to approach the effort that can offer a better result, and they are available to everyone.

The Go Cogno Credo is a set of simple concepts to help guide you on your way. I encourage you to study them, internalize them and apply them to your actions.

G — Grind it out

When I think of the people I have seen halt or reverse their cognitive loss, each of them went about it in their own quiet way.

They were regular people who led ordinary lives. They didn't wear a cape, or leap tall buildings in a single bound. But they were heroic enough to take on MCI and if there was a superpower they brought to the battle, it was their sheer relentlessness.

Getting to a place of better brain health can be a grind. It takes effort, but even more, it asks for that effort to be sustained over a period of months, or even years.

You didn't go to bed one night with normal cognition and wake up the next morning with MCI. It was a long time coming. And the undoing of it can be equally arduous.

It's not that it can't be done. It's definitely possible to slow, halt or reverse cognitive decline. And in rare cases, it might even happen quickly.

But not often.

Usually, it's a long, slow road. From my experience, those who understand that going in, and approach the journey with patience and perseverance, are the ones who most often seem to prevail.

O — Orient yourself toward action

There are things you can take for better brain health. Certain medications or supplements may be appropriate for you, and if your doctor recommends them, then by all means, take them.

But for the treatment of MCI, there aren't a whole lot of things you can "take." On the other hand, there are plenty of things you can "do." And they work.

Someday, we'll have better medical treatments. But here's what I want to impress upon you: The lifestyle choices I've spent the last few chapters talking about — physical activity, diet, stress, sleep, brain training — already offer a benefit that medicine may never be able to match.

And they're available right now. They can be the difference-maker for you. So put your emphasis there.

Here's an exercise that may help. Divide a piece of paper down the middle. On one side, list the things you are taking. On the other, list the things you are doing. Ideally, the list of things you're doing should be at least as long as the list of things you're taking, if not longer.

The way to go aggressively after your MCI is less in the taking than in the doing. Take what you're told to take, but define yourself by what you do.

C — Compound your way to a better outcome

You need to make changes in your life, and you need to make them stick. By turning them into habits — behaviors so ingrained into your life that you do them automatically. Like brushing your teeth or having your morning coffee.

But with health behavior change, success depends on how you approach it.

The wrong way is the "New Year's resolution" method, where you set out with the best of intentions, but you fail because your goal was too vague or too ambitious. So don't do that. Do what works instead.

The right way to get results is by making small, behavior-specific changes one week at a time. Don't say, "I'm going to get more exercise." Instead, say, "Tomorrow, I'm going to walk once around the block." And then gradually increase from there.

Don't say, "I'm going to give up soda." Instead, say, "I'm going to drink one less soda every day and replace it with a bottle of kombucha." Then you lock in that habit and continue to cut back a little more each week.

These changes may seem small, but they add up. They compound, the same way interest compounds on money you put in the bank.

In fact, that analogy is a perfect way to think about it. You're determined to save your brain, right? So here's what you do. You open a cognitive savings account, and you start making regular deposits into

117

it. Those deposits are in the form of small changes in health behavior, which you sustain and turn into habits. You earn compounding interest on your deposits, and over time the dividend can be a better cognitive outcome.

In the real world, that's how health behavior change happens. Commit to the process and start making those modest weekly deposits. That's what'll pay off for you in the long run.

O — Optimize for maximum benefit

Exercise? Brain training? Adopting the MIND Diet? What you choose to do is up to you. But whatever you undertake, go all in. Don't settle for doing the least amount you can get away with. Optimize it for the maximum benefit.

That is one of the biggest differences between the way the average person approaches brain health, and the way someone with MCI needs to approach it.

You need to be more aggressive. You need to leverage it for all it's worth. Not right away. It's fine to start at a more moderate level. But begin with the end in mind, and work your way up.

Take meditation, for instance. The ideal is 20 minutes a day. If you're new to meditation, it's OK to start out by meditating for 2 minutes a day. But let 20 minutes be your eventual goal and keep adding minutes until you get there.

Do the same for anything else you decide to work on. You don't have to try everything and you don't have to do anything perfectly. But whatever you put your oomph into, give your brain the maximum benefit it has to offer.

G — Go with your gut

Where do I begin? How do I even get started?

Every person with mild cognitive impairment confronts that question at some point. You know you need to do something. You have to start somewhere. But the challenge is so enormous. And there's so much at stake. And so many choices. It can be overwhelming.

So let's keep it simple.

You are the right person to make that choice, and the way to decide is by trusting your gut.

That's what I learned from Dr. Kate Lorig, and she ought to know.

Dr. Lorig is a Stanford University public health expert who's spent nearly four decades researching and developing strategies to help people improve health habits and manage chronic illnesses. Her book , *Living a Healthy Life with Chronic Conditions*, has sold more than one million copies.

Over the years, Dr. Lorig has become a believer in the power of letting people determine their own goals. She says people have a feel for what they need to work on first, and their instincts are usually spot on.

"I can't judge what's important to somebody," she says. "I trust in people making good decisions about where they start. I really believe very strongly in self-tailoring and the wisdom of the individual."

Of course, using the assessment tools in Chapter 4 can help. And you want to listen to the advice of your doctor.

But the decision is yours, and you are eminently qualified to make it. Don't overthink it. Let your intuition guide you, pick something you feel ready to do and GET TO IT!!!! It'll be the right choice. The only wrong choice would be not to get started at all.

N — Know your numbers

Our brain isn't something we carry around in a glass jar under our arm. It's part of our body. Brain health is integral to heart health and overall health. So it's essential to cognition that you get regular health checkups and manage your blood pressure, cholesterol, blood sugar level and other key health indicators.

We know that untreated high blood pressure, also known as hypertension, is one of the biggest risk factors for MCI and increases the risk of progressing to dementia. It's estimated that nearly half of all adults in the United States have high blood pressure, yet only 24 percent of them have it under control. For anyone with MCI, it is absolutely essential to have your blood pressure checked regularly and keep it in a healthy range, through medication and healthy habits.

The other basics of heart health also apply to brain health. Don't smoke. "Know your numbers" for cholesterol, blood sugar and body mass index, and work with your doctor to get and keep them in a healthy range. If you have diabetes, managing it is vital. The risk of dementia is so connected to diabetes that some neurologists refer to Alzheimer's as "Type 3 diabetes."

This is all basic stuff, but it's so important. Address any of these essential health indicators, and the benefit will go directly to your brain.

O — Overindulge in self-care

Now is the time to put yourself first. You need to be good to you, both in the words you say to yourself and in the ways you treat yourself.

One thing I encourage people with MCI to do is count how many minutes they devote every day to self-care, and then increase that amount of time by two minutes every day for a month. But not activities of empty diversion. Things that nourish your well-being.

Music. Affirmation. Meditation. Journaling. Gratitude. Prayer. Poetry. Love-making. A hearty laugh. A glass of red wine. A walk in the woods. A letter to a friend. Let these be a healing balm in your life.

To get well, treat yourself well.

THE GO COGNO CREDO IN SUMMARY

You can improve your chances of slowing, halting or reversing MCI when you

- **G — Grind it out**
- **O — Orient yourself toward action**
- **C — Compound your way to a better outcome**
- **O — Optimize for maximum benefit**
- **G — Go with your gut**
- **N — Know your numbers**
- **O — Overindulge in self-care**

ONE ACTION, RIGHT NOW: Count the number of minutes you spend in self-care today, and then tomorrow, add two additional minutes of self-care to your daily routine.

I WANT MY MIND BACK

CHAPTER 17 — Time To Go Cogno!

NOW BEGINS the journey.

You are ready to be an advocate for your own care, and the architect of your own actions.

And what you do next isn't really all that important. What matters right now is the simple act of doing it. Getting started.

When we look at a broad general population of people who have been diagnosed with mild cognitive impairment, we know that most of them — and by most, I mean close to 90 percent — will either see their MCI stabilize or reverse over a period of four to five years.

That's across everyone who has MCI, and those are good odds. With a diagnosis to act upon, the right doctor, a good grasp of your own unique vulnerabilities, and a willingness to address them, you give yourself an even better chance.

Cognitive impairment can be slowed, halted or reversed when caught at the earliest stages.

Two or three years ago, no one was saying that, and that message still hasn't caught up with much of the medical community. Too many doctors remain stuck in "not-much-we-can-do" mode.

Fortunately, there are doctors who know better and can help you do better.

One of them is Dr. Mary Kay Ross, whom we met in Chapter 14. She calls MCI "type 2 diabetes for the brain."

"I feel if you bring me someone with type 2 diabetes, there's no reason for that person to be a type 2 diabetic; I can fix it," says Dr. Ross, CEO of the Brain Health & Research Institute in Seattle. "MCI is the same way. We can definitely halt the progression of the disease and restore cognition.

"With MCI, we don't know how long it took to get there, but the disease is a response to something," she says. "If we can get you when you're really early MCI, then honestly it just becomes a matter of doing a deep dive to find out what is causing the person's disease and undo it."

IT'S JUST YOU AND YOUR MCI

These days, doctors who truly understand the nature of mild cognitive impairment are allowed to say that. The scientific evidence proves it, and so do the results they're seeing with people who have MCI. People like you.

But don't misunderstand how such results are achieved. These doctors, smart and dedicated though they are, don't get those results. Their patients do.

The doctor guides, but the patient does the work. When I look at the people whom I have seen halt or reverse their MCI, what strikes me most is how much of that they achieved on their own.

They had good, capable medical care and took full advantage of it. But there is only so much a neurologist can do for you.

Even in the case of a sophisticated, highly individualized treatment plan, the doctor will typically give you things to "take" — some combination of medication and/or supplements — and things to "do" — exercise, dietary changes, stress reduction, etc. And then they send you on your way.

Once you get home, for the next six months, or the next year, it's just you and your MCI. And either you're getting the better of it, or it's getting the better of you.

The people I have seen get the better of their MCI are the ones who chose to Go Cogno on it. They took their cognitive health into their own hands, and a fair amount of what they did, they figured out for themselves.

Your journey will be different than their journey, and you will have to navigate your own way through it. What science tells us is that the people with MCI who tend to do better are the ones who

- get their body moving,
- clean up their diet,
- manage their stress,
- get a good night's sleep, and
- do brain training.

If one of those is a glaring vulnerability for you, that would be a fine place to start. Or you may choose to start somewhere else. You're the best one to decide that.

There is no one formula, and no right or perfect place to begin. There will be some trial and error. You will learn along the way. As you do, remember the words of Tolkien, who said: "Not all those who wander are lost."

What you need to do will become clearer to you as you progress. Whatever you try, make sure it's safe and has real scientific evidence behind it. You don't have to do everything right. You only have to do enough to tip the cognitive balance back your way.

At some point in the journey, whether right away or later on, you will have to come to terms with whatever your "No. 1" is — that thing that was one too many hits for your brain to absorb and tipped the balance against you. Most likely, it won't be the only thing you need to address. But your ability to slow, halt or reverse your cognitive decline will be compromised until you identify and disarm it.

A WIN IS A WIN IS A WIN

I'm always careful how I talk about dementia to a readership that has mild cognitive impairment. Alzheimer's is their greatest fear, and MCI puts them at greater risk for it. But for the majority of people with cognitive impairment, the cause is something other than Alzheimer's.

For them, the underlying cause could be any number of things, most of which are treatable. Address it, and your cognition can improve.

For those who have a confirmed diagnosis of MCI due to Alzheimer's, or who have been told the likely cause is Alzheimer's, the prognosis is different, but the approach is the same. Either way, you want to go after your MCI early and aggressively. Even people presumed to have underlying Alzheimer's can potentially slow the progression at the MCI stage by adopting healthy habits.

Dr. Joel Salinas, a neurologist at Massachusetts General Hospital, tells the *Harvard Health Letter* that he sees people "stay in the MCI stage for many years, even when we presume it was a neurodegenerative disease . . . The people who spend the most time cognitively stable are often the ones who stick to lifestyle recommendations."

Your cognition is worth defending. If you slow it down, that's a win. If you halt it, that's a win. If you reverse it and return to cognitively normal, even if only for some period of time, that's a win.

In your mind, you may be saying, "If I could reverse this, that would be the ultimate win." I encourage people not to think that way. A win is a win. Yes, it is possible to reverse MCI, and it does sometimes happen, but it's not the most likely outcome.

The University of Pittsburgh study that followed nearly 900 people with MCI found that 35 percent of them either reverted to cognitively normal or fluctuated between MCI and cognitively normal over a period of five years.

The more common result was for people to stabilize their MCI. More than half were able to do that. That's worth shooting for, and given how often it's achieved, a realistic ambition.

SIX FACTORS THAT LEND TO REVERSING MCI

That was Miriam's modest goal at the start of her journey, if you recall. She did not set out with any expectation of reversing her MCI. All she wanted was to stop it from getting worse. She was able to do more than that, partly because she did the right things and did them emphatically, but also because she was a prime candidate for it.

The recent explosion in research around mild cognitive impairment includes an important mega-study that considered the cognitive out-comes of nearly 7,000 people with MCI. The results, published in the *International Journal of Geriatric Psychiatry*, found there are six factors that make someone more likely to return to cognitively normal. They are

- being of a younger age.
- having a higher level of education.
- having higher scores on cognitive tests like the MMSE.
- not having the APOE4 gene.
- not having hypertension (or having it and being treated for it).
- not having a history of stroke.

If you look at Miriam, she checks most of those boxes. So she had certain advantages as she began her effort. I expect you are measuring yourself against that list, and perhaps you do, too. If so, use that as further motivation to take on your MCI and go after it resolutely.

If you don't, please understand these are not prerequisites. Slowing, halting or reversing MCI is a possibility no matter what your age, level of education or genetic status, as long as you are willing to do the work.

Let's say you set the same goal Miriam did. Your goal is to halt your cognitive loss. So you Go Cogno.

You begin in fits and starts, just trying to find your way. But then you gradually hone in on some things that seem to be working, and stick with them, and try a few more things. And all the time you're keeping a close eye on your percentile score in BrainHQ, and it's holding steady, and the next time you see the neurologists, it's good news. You've stabilized your MCI. And then you manage to keep it stable, for three or four or five years, or maybe for many years after that.

What would that mean in your life? What would you do with that blessing?

"DOES ANYONE KNOW . . . . ?"

That's the question I asked a woman with MCI who has become a colleague and friend of mine. Her name is Cheryl Stevenson. She is 62 years old and lives by herself in a small town in rural New Hampshire.

Cheryl began noticing cognitive problems while she was still in her 40s. But rather than ignore the problem and live in denial, she went to see a doctor, who told her the one thing she didn't want to hear. She had Alzheimer's. Or so the doctor said.

Cheryl decided to get a second opinion. She was evaluated by another specialist, and he changed the diagnosis to mild cognitive impairment. She had no idea what that was. Back then, information about MCI was nearly nonexistent.

So Cheryl struggled to understand what she was dealing with, but one thing was clear. She had to make changes in her life. And this wasn't going to be about getting a gym membership or going vegan. Cheryl was in an abusive relationship. The neurologist told her that if she didn't get out of that situation, the relentless stress would continue to take a toll on her cognition in a way that nothing else could undo. She knew he was right.

It took courage, but Cheryl escaped that relationship and built a new life for herself. Her MCI came along with her, but she has found a peace and acceptance that allows her to cope with it.

Back in 2017 she wrote eloquently about her MCI in a poem called "Does Anyone Know?"

"Does anyone know the frustration that I feel when I can't remember something?" she asks. "Does anyone know how much I wish my brain functioned normally?"

But she has a spirit and resilience that allow her to push through the down moments.

"I'm still here, I'm just different," she says. "I can't choose what I remember and what I forget, but this memory impairment that I live with does not define who I am. Does anyone know that I am still ME?"

MCI is what Cheryl has. It's not who she is. She continues to find in her life a meaning and joy that MCI cannot take away from her, and that is even more true now that she is a grandparent.

One day, in particular, drove that home poignantly. Cheryl would share the story later in a Facebook post that brought tears to my eyes. I can't improve upon her telling of it, so I'll let you read it in her own words:

"Today my daughter & son-in-law had to work & the daycare was closed. A few days ago, when she told me, I told her I could babysit in the morning until around 12 noon. This morning, after I arrived at their house, a few minutes later they left for work. Before they left, my daughter showed me a note on the counter explaining when the babies should need bottles, naps & cereal etc. They were still sleeping when I arrived. I had a fun day with my almost 10-month-old twin granddaughters! Everything went well & no problems at all. I feel so blessed to have these babies in my life! I think that I was there for almost 5 hours & I think this is the longest time that I have babysat them. I'm so glad that their parents feel that I can handle this. Yay, me!"

I picture Cheryl spending the morning so lovingly and capably caring for two 10-month-old babies. And then I picture that same woman some 15 years ago, sitting panic-stricken in a doctor's office, having just been informed, "You have Alzheimer's."

Had her worst fears come true, Cheryl would not have lived long enough to see her granddaughters, or if she had, she would not have known who they were. But her fears were not her fate. She chose a different future for herself. She chose to defend her cognition.

SMALL STEPS, WELL WITHIN YOUR CAPABILITIES

Someone with mild cognitive impairment today has so many advantages that Cheryl didn't. Back when she was diagnosed, that feels like the Stone Age of MCI treatment. There is so much more a doctor can do for you now, and so much you can do for yourself.

None of that will happen on its own. You have to make it happen, but you are highly motivated, and what you need to do is well within your capabilities.

There are changes you need to make. You will succeed by breaking that down into one small, simple step after another, each of which you are ready to attempt and feel confident you can accomplish.

How hard will that be? Let me ask you this: How hard was it to buy and read this book? That's your answer. It wasn't hard at all. It's what you were ready to do, and you did it. The next thing you need to do won't require any more effort than this one did.

Take your inspiration from others before you who have managed to halt or reverse their cognitive decline. They didn't approach it any differently than you are. They educated themselves. And they took action, one day at a time. That's it. That's how it's done. Are you capable of doing what they did? No need to even ask. You're already doing it.

What's required to effect change in your life is something you've already summoned. You have it within you. And now you're going to turn it loose. You're going to unleash it on your MCI.

Yay, you!

What's Next?

Congratulations, and welcome to what's next. You have come to the end of this book and the beginning of your journey. So where do you go from here?

That's for you to choose. But as you prepare to get started, please let me express my gratitude. I want to thank you for buying and reading my book. I know you had plenty of other choices, but you picked this book and for that I am grateful.

If you found this book helpful, I would love to hear from you. Please consider posting a candid review on Amazon. Your honest feedback helps me reach more people, so I can serve them too, and allows me to continue to make this book better. If you're willing to leave a review, you can do that by clicking here.

Next, I have an invitation for you. Two invitations, actually.

First, I invite you to take the "Make Your Brain" Healthy Eating Challenge. For someone determined to defend their cognition, this is the ideal starter kit.

The challenge is a guided exercise that offers you an all-important, early win against MCI. At the same time, it gets you into the habit of developing better health habits, so you can keep right on setting goals and achieving them.

And I don't want you to have to do any of this alone. So my second special invitation is for you to join our private Facebook community, a safe, welcoming place where people with MCI gather to support each other's efforts and succeed together. I hope to see you there.

Take the "Make Your Brain" Healthy Eating Challenge

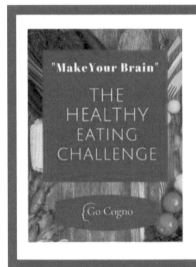

"Whatever you eat will either break the brain or make the brain."

— Dr. Ayesha Sherzai

Want your mind back? Food is a fine place to start. What we put on our plate can savage cognition — or salvage it. This challenge will change your diet for good.

This simple, two-week challenge will help improve your diet in ways that make your brain healthier, more resilient, and better able to fend off MCI. It's designed to:

- Show you what foods you need to eat more (or less) of, and exactly how much is the right amount for optimal brain health.
- Give you the tools to make healthy changes in your diet, and turn them into lasting habits.

Sign up for the "Make Your Brain" Healthy Eating Challenge today, and change your diet for good.

Take the Challenge here — gocogno.com/myb-challenge

Join our private Facebook community

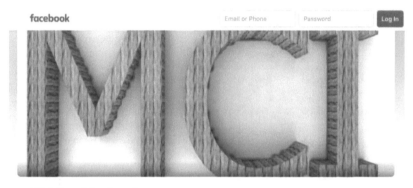

Mild Cognitive Impairment
🔒 Private group · 1.1K members

Mild cognitive impairment can be a lonely, isolating condition. It's easy to feel like you are the only person who has MCI, and no one else understands what you're going through.

So please know this. You are not alone. The Go Cogno community includes thousands of people in the United States and across the globe who are living with MCI and supporting each other in that shared human experience.

That is why I'm issuing you this special invitation to join our private Facebook group for people with mild cognitive impairment. This group is a safe, confidential, welcoming place where members offer each other comfort, support and encouragement.

Have a burning question you're trying to get answered? Need a kind word to lift your spirits? Have a small victory, a humorous anecdote or an inspirational quote you'd like to share? Our MCI group is the place for you. Use the link below to go to our private Facebook page and ask to join. We look forward to welcoming you in open arms.

Ask to join here — gocogno.com/mci-group

APPENDIX A — Frequently Asked Questions

Mild cognitive impairment is not a disease, and it's not a form of dementia. Rather, it's a medical term for a degree of cognitive loss that is outside the normal range for someone your age but not debilitating.

There are two forms of mild cognitive impairment. With amnestic MCI, the primary symptom is a loss of memory. When other types of thinking skills are affected, that's called non-amnestic MCI.

Here are answers to some frequently asked questions about MCI.

Q. How common is MCI?

A. For people over the age of 65, it's estimated that somewhere between 15 and 20 percent have mild cognitive impairment. The risk continues to go up as we age.

Q. What are the signs of MCI?

A. Common symptoms of mild cognitive impairment include

- experiencing forgetfulness often enough that it worries you.
- struggling to understand or remember information you read.
- a decline in ability to plan things or solve problems.
- not being able to follow a conversation that's occurring around you.

- having a supervisor or co-workers express concern over a decline in performance on the job.
- repeating a question over and over.
- forgetting the name of a family member.
- losing interest in favorite activities.
- getting lost in a familiar setting.
- floundering at tasks that used to be routine, like paying bills.
- showing poor judgment or struggling to make decisions.
- difficulty finding the right words.
- family or friends are expressing concerns about your memory.

Q. How can a doctor tell if I have MCI?

A. A proper diagnosis of MCI is arrived at through a process that includes a medical workup, a review of your medical history, lab tests, an assessment of daily functions, the observations of family or friends, and a neurological exam. (See more details in Appendix B.)

Q. If I have MCI, does that mean I'm going to get dementia?

A. In some cases, MCI is a "pre-dementia" condition. "This means that the brain diseases that cause dementia are already established," according to the Alzheimer's Society. However, a diagnosis of MCI does not necessarily mean the underlying cause is Alzheimer's or some other form of dementia. There are many other possible causes of MCI.

Q. Can a doctor tell if my mild cognitive impairment is an early stage of Alzheimer's?

A. Science has made great strides in the early detection of Alzheimer's.

The beta-amyloid "plaques" associated with Alzheimer's begin to build up in the brain a decade or more before people show any symptoms of the disease. It's now possible to identify amyloid accumulations in the brain, using a special scan called an amyloid PET scan or by analyzing cerebrospinal fluid. However, these tests are expensive and invasive and in many cases not covered by insurance, so people with MCI may not have access to these tests. Researchers are working on simple, less expensive ways to detect Alzheimer's, such as a blood test, and that may become available within a few years.

Q. If it's not dementia, what other conditions can lead to MCI, and is there anything I can do about them?

A. There are many other potential causes. Sleep apnea and depression are two possible culprits. Both are strongly associated with cognitive problems, and experts say it's important to be evaluated for them. Memory loss also can be caused by such factors as a thyroid condition, a vitamin deficiency or adverse side effects from one or more medications. Cognitive decline also has been linked to diabetes, hypertension or other chronic conditions. If you aren't getting physical exercise or a healthy amount of social or mental stimulation, that can dim cognition as well. The good news is that these are treatable problems. If any of these is identified as contributing to cognitive loss, it can be addressed.

Q. What are the chances that my cognition can improve?

A. Experts say that depends on a complex set of factors unique to you and your situation. There is no one set of odds for everyone; it varies widely.

Researchers at the University of Pittsburgh followed nearly 900 adults with mild cognitive impairment over a period of five years, to see how they fared.

The results, published in the *Journal of the American Geriatrics Society*, showed that

- 53 percent stabilized at MCI.
- 35 percent reverted to cognitively normal or fluctuated between MCI and normal cognition.
- 12 percent progressed to dementia.

Q. Are there any medicines I can take for MCI?

A. There's not an FDA-approved medication for MCI. If the cause of your memory loss is a treatable condition, your doctor may prescribe one or more medicines as part of a treatment plan. Often, lifestyle changes will be part of that plan as well. It's also important to understand that cognitive decline sometimes results from taking inappropriate medications. In such cases, less medication — not more — may be the answer. Your doctor may decide it's best to gradually wean you off those drugs.

If your MCI is a pre-dementia condition, there are currently no drugs approved by the FDA to treat people at the stage of mild cognitive impairment. Physicians do have some latitude in prescribing drugs "off-label" and may choose to give a patient with MCI a drug approved for the treatment of Alzheimer's or other conditions. Meanwhile, many potential drugs are being studied right now, and clinical trials may involve patients with mild cognitive impairment as well as Alzheimer's patients.

Q. How about alternative treatments for MCI?

A. Here's what the Mayo Clinic says about that:

"Some supplements — including vitamin E, ginkgo and others — have been purported to help prevent or delay the progression of mild cognitive impairment. However, no supplement has shown any benefit in a clinical trial."

Q. If there's not a medicine I can take for it, is there something else I can do to slow down my mental decline?

A. A significant body of scientific evidence tells us that lifestyle choices can improve brain health and reduce the risk of cognitive decline. These include not smoking, managing blood pressure and cholesterol, being physically active, eating a healthy diet, getting enough sleep and keeping yourself mentally and socially stimulated.

The book *Living with Mild Cognitive Impairment* says for someone with MCI, adopting better health habits can make a difference. It says:

"Undoubtedly, it is better to have led a healthy lifestyle throughout your life, but there is good reason to believe that it is never too late to start. We advise our clients and you to make these positive healthy and lifestyle changes now. Research has shown our lifestyle choices can have a real impact on our physical and cognitive health that could prevent or delay the onset of dementia for those at risk."

APPENDIX B — A Proper Diagnosis

What does a proper diagnosis of mild cognitive impairment look like? The American Academy of Neurology offers good guidance on that part of its official MCI treatment guidelines.

This is what the ANA says should take place when a patient expresses concerns about memory or other cognitive problems:

STEP 1 — The doctor should assess the patient for mild cognitive impairment, rather than dismiss the problem as a result of normal aging.

STEP 2 — That assessment should not be based solely on the concerns the patient and/or family are expressing. The doctor should give the patient some form of brief, validated memory test.
   Among the tests a doctor might use for that are:

- Montreal Cognitive Assessment (MoCA) — Known to be particularly sensitive to detecting MCI
- Mini-Mental State Exam (MMSE) – Sensitivity to MCI is low, only 18 percent
- Mini-Cog – Takes only one to three minutes to administer
- St. Louis University Mental Status (SLUMS)

STEP 3 — A patient who scores in the range of MCI on a preliminary test should be given more in-depth testing, such as a neuropsychological exam. A diagnosis of MCI should be based on this more thorough testing and examination, not solely on the score of a preliminary test.

STEP 4 — If a thorough exam indicates mild cognitive impairment, the doctor should take care to determine whether the proper diagnosis is MCI or dementia. This is determined by giving the patient what is called a "functional" assessment to gauge how well the patient is able to independently perform daily tasks.

STEP 5 — Unless the doctor is well versed in treating cognitive impairment, a patient diagnosed with MCI should be referred to a specialist who has that expertise, such as a neurologist, internist or geriatrician.

APPENDIX C — Other Books To Read

Now that you have read my book, you have an introduction into what MCI is and how it can potentially be slowed, halted or reversed.

But I encourage you to keep going. There is still so much opportunity to deepen your understanding of this condition you are experiencing, and add to your arsenal of ways to defend against it.

I'm reminded of the words of Pema Chodron, who said: "Nothing ever goes away until it has taught us what we need to know."

There is more you need to know about MCI than can be contained in a single book. So keep learning. Read more. And read these three books in particular. I consider them the three absolute "must-reads" for anyone with mild cognitive impairment. What they can add to your understanding of MCI is invaluable.

Living With Mild Cognitive Impairment: A Guide to Maximizing Brain Health and Reducing the Risk of Dementia
  By Nicole D. Anderson, Kelly J. Murphy and Angela K. Troyer

This classic book on mild cognitive impairment was years ahead of its time when it was published in 2012. The authors run a world-class program for MCI patients at Baycrest in Toronto and this seminal work combines the best elements of a medical explainer with a helpful "how-to" approach. The guidance it offers on coping with MCI is particularly strong, and the chapter on memory compensation techniques can be life-changing all by itself.

The Alzheimer's Solution: A Breakthrough Program to Prevent and Reverse the Symptoms of Cognitive Decline at Every Age
   By Drs. Dean & Ayesha Sherzai

When I recommend this book to people, they sometimes ask, "Why should I read this? I don't have Alzheimer's. I have MCI." I tell them, "That's the whole point. This isn't a book about Alzheimer's. This is a book about how not to get Alzheimer's." Drs. Dean and Ayesha Sherzai are doing pioneering work, and their practice focuses on people with MCI because they believe "that population is most amenable to reversing." The chapter on diet and nutrition is exceptional, and stories they tell throughout the book offer example after example of how real people were able to halt or reverse their cognitive loss. The eight-page assessment tool at the end of Chapter 2 is a wonderful bonus.

The End of Alzheimer's: The First Program to Prevent and Reverse Cognitive Decline
   By Dr. Dale E. Bredesen

Dr. Dale Bredesen is a controversial figure who has many admirers and just as many detractors. You are free to form your own opinion about his approach, but if you've been diagnosed with MCI, you need to read this book. What he teaches is too important to ignore, and even if you decide the "Bredesen protocol" is not for you, there are many elements of it that you can incorporate on your own. I truly believe his concept of a "cognoscopy" represents the future of MCI treatment for those who are not making the progress they want through lifestyle changes and traditional medical care.

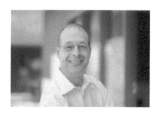

About the Author

Tony Dearing is the founder and publisher of GoCogno.com, the website for people with mild cognitive impairment. His interest in the subject arose from a deeply personal place. His mother had MCI, progressed to dementia and died in 2014. As the journalist in the family, it fell upon him to write her obituary. And he kept on writing. The following year, Dearing launched his award-winning column on brain health and the prevention of dementia for NJ.com and the *Star-Ledger* in New Jersey.

Yet even as he emerged as a leading writer on the subject of Alzheimer's, he saw a great, unmet need among the millions of older Americans who are being diagnosed with mild cognitive impairment. He felt drawn to serve them out of what he describes as a journalistic "sense of wonder."

"I wondered why I couldn't find accurate, up-to-date information on MCI," he says. "I wondered why no one was writing about it. Finally, I wondered, why not me?" He launched GoCogno.com in 2017, and the timing proved prescient. Over the next two years, a series of advances in research and treatment led experts to begin talking about Alzheimer's as preventable and MCI as reversible.

Dearing continues to publish articles and videos on the latest developments in cognitive care, but his greater goal is to bring that information into the real world and help people with MCI defend their cognition through health behavior change. He finds that real progress occurs when you "meet people where they are and help them take the next step forward."

Dearing resides in New Jersey, where he works as Director of News Operations for NJ Advance Media. Prior to that, he spent much of his career in print journalism, serving as editor of two daily newspapers in Michigan. He scrupulously attends to his own brain health through a regimen that includes morning walks with his wife, Pei-Pei, swimming, a healthy diet, meditation, yoga, brain training, journaling, daily affirmations and cultural activities. He is always willing to try something new, except TikTok, which he doesn't understand at all and hopes is just a fad that will go away as soon as possible.

The author welcomes your thoughts, suggestions or questions about this book or about brain health in general.
Email him at: tonydearing@gocogno.com

You can connect with me on:
🌐 https://gocogno.com

Made in United States
Troutdale, OR
01/27/2024

17143988R00090